The Limits of Professional Power

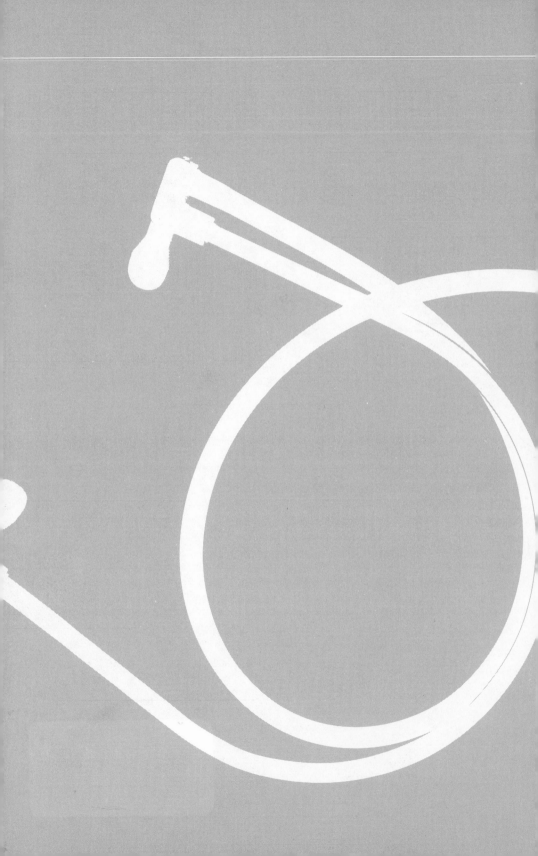

The Limits of Professional Power

National Health Care in the Federal Republic of Germany

Deborah A. Stone

The University of Chicago Press
Chicago and London

To Dr. Joseph L. Lewis
whose care for me in childhood and beyond
remains my standard for health services
and to Dr. Manfred Pflanz whose warmth, humor
and knowledge helped keep my research in the
perspective of life's true pleasures

DEBORAH A. STONE is associate professor of
political science at the Massachusetts Institute
of Technology.

The University of Chicago Press, Chicago 60637
The University of Chicago Press, Ltd., London

Library of Congress Cataloging in Publication Data

Stone, Deborah A.
   The limits of professional power.

   Bibliography: p.
   Includes index.
   1. Medical policy—Germany, West. 2. Medical
care—Germany, West. 3. Physicians—Germany, West.
4. Insurance, Health—Germany, West. 5. Power
(Social sciences) I. Title. [DNLM: 1. Insurance,
Health—Germany, West. 2 State medicine—Germany, West.
3. Physicians—Germany, West. W275 GG4 S8L]
RA395.G4S76   362.1'042   80–16864
ISBN 0–226–77553–4

Contents

Figures

Tables

If you are at all like me, you turned to the preface first, in the hopes of catching a glimpse of the person inside the author. The person inside this author is still somewhat of a mystery to me, but I don't need to tell you that a preface is just a thinly disguised excuse for fond reminiscence, anyway.

To this day, when people ask me how I got interested in West German national health insurance, I still cannot give a coherent answer. It was certainly *not*, as I imply in the book, because the West German health system offered the right combination of characteristics to study the theoretical questions I had set for myself. More probably, it had to do with my lifelong fascination with medicine (kindled by my teenage TV hero, Ben Casey), my insatiable desire to experience foreign cultures (inherited from my grandmother, no doubt), and my yen for learning foreign languages (German happened to be next on my list at the time). As it turned out, the research topic satisfied all these parts of me and was theoretically interesting besides.

In 1972–73, I was a visiting scholar at the Max Planck Institut zur Erforschung der Lebensbedingungen der wissenschaftlich-technischen Welt, in Starnberg. (A title, by the way, that I learned to roll easily off my tongue, which feat was proof enough for my mother that I deserved a Ph.D.). To Jürgen Habermas, director of the Institute, and the staff and colleagues there, I am grateful for the help and camaraderie I received. Claus Offe was a wonderful colleague and friend that year—and still is—and I always cherish a chance to talk politics with him.

My German colleagues let their special national gift of *Gastfreundlichkeit* blur the edges between work and friendship. Christa Altensletter, Manfred and Elizabeth Pflanz, Ulrich and Christiane Geissler, Claus and Sabine Offe, Prof. and Mrs. Christian von Ferber, and Peter and Irma Nippert all shared their knowledge of health policy and their loves and hates of things German. Some of my favorite moments in "conducting my research" comprised bedtime stories with Julia Offe, flute and cello duets with Sebastian Pflanz, a puppet show written and produced by Matthias and Jani Pflanz, country excursions and fine meals with Peter, Irma, and Easy Nippert, and many long lunches of *gelbe Rüben* with the Von Ferbers.

Ulrich Geissler deserves to be called the patron saint of this study. I first met him when he was assigned (or so I presume—he never told me) to answer my rather naive inquiry to the Minister of Labor in 1971. He might have treated me as another interruption in his day, but from the very first meeting, he took my research seriously and was personally concerned that I should truly understand the German system and its problems. Since then, he has helped me in a thousand ways. He arranged interviews with officials in numerous agencies, practically served as my travel agent in West Germany, let me loose in the library of the Bundesverband der Ortskrankenkassen and then in its xerox room, and provided a personal reference service over the years by sending me articles, documents, and reports as they appeared. Most important, he has spent hours with me explaining, discussing, questioning, and answering.

Every project also has its guardian angel, and I was lucky to have a few. The Center for European Studies at Harvard University gave me a grant to explore some preliminary ideas and later, an office in which to sort them out and write them down. The Deutscher Akademischer Austauschdienst gave me a scholarship to study German at the Goethe Institute in Iserlohn. There I partook of absolutely inspired teaching and the most creative improvisational approach to language learning on the part of my classmates from all over the world. The German Marshall Fund of the United States gave me a postdoctoral fellowship that enabled me to return to Germany for an extensive research trip and then to spend several months writing a book. I was honored to be present at the reception where then Chancellor Willy Brandt presented the endowment for the German Marshall Fund in 1973, and since that time, I have seen the fund stimulate and support some wonderful research on common problems of advanced industrial societies. Peter Weitz of the German Marshall Fund was especially helpful as an intellectual matchmaker among scholars of Western Europe.

I hope some of my former teachers and present colleagues at MIT will find a little of themselves in this book. Suzanne Berger taught the one thing most worth teaching—how to ask questions—and she taught it in the best possible way—by example. Mike Lipsky taught me to look at policy as the outcome of discretionary decisions of service providers, and helped me find some creative paths around my own mental blocks. Marty Rein first pointed out the issue of professional accountability as one worthy of study, and approached it with his inimitable style of making up "stories" from dry research data. Harvey Sapolsky treated me as a colleague from the day I first asked him to join my thesis committee, and his substantive suggestions and general concern have always made me feel lucky to be in his orbit.

Christa Altenstetter, Suzanne Berger, Ulrich Geissler, Arnold

Heidenheimer, Joe Lipscomb, Mike Lipsky, Ted Marmor, Manfred Pflanz, Peter Rosenberg, Harvey Sapolsky and Prof. von Ferber all read drafts of the manuscript and gave extensive and thoughtful comments. My father also read drafts and spared me extensive comments, but gave me lots of appreciation and encouragement instead. If any large errors remain, I won't blame any of them, but I do hope they will each feel morally obligated to buy me a hot fudge sundae as consolation. Chuck Lockman, Mark Gittelman, and Norma Kriger all provided help with typing, editing, and proofreading the manuscript. If any small errors remain, I hope they will feel similarly obligated, though I would settle for a cone—with jimmies.

Randy Bovbjerg participated in this study in more ways than he probably cares to remember. Of all of them, I will always treasure most his unfailing moral support.

The Nature, Sources, and Limits of Physicians' Power | Chapter One

The Nature of Physicians' Power

Although there is widespread agreement that physicians constitute one of the most powerful groups in modern industrial societies, we actually have very little understanding of the nature of their power. Most scholars would agree that there is something unique about the medical profession, or perhaps about all professions, that renders them a special elite. But beyond the commonplace observations that professionals tend to have a lot of wealth and a lot of prestige, there have been few attempts to specify more precisely what kinds of decisions and resources physicians actually control.[1]

One of the best efforts is Eliot Freidson's *Profession of Medicine.*[2] Freidson argues that "autonomy of technique," or control over the content of one's own work, is the most important distinguishing characteristic of professions as compared with other occupations. He goes on to argue that this autonomy of technique gives professions a wedge into other "zones" of practice; in the case of medicine, control over technique is broadened to include control over facilities, organization of service delivery, and training.[3] Freidson also points out that the extent to which autonomy is generalized beyond the technical aspects of work varies in different societies. In the Soviet Union, for instance, the state controls many areas of health policy that are left to the medical profession in the United States.

The concept of autonomy is useful and suggests a baisc difference in the political position of professions and other occupations. The concept does not, however, distinguish between the collective and the individual dimensions of physicians' power, a distinction that would seem to be very important. In any discussion of physicians' power, one wants to be clear about the difference between the power of the individual physician (with respect to his patients, the state, other physicians, or employers, for example) and the power of physicians as a group (with respect to the state, or other interest groups, for example).

The role of physicians in policymaking has been fairly widely studied under the rubric of interest group politics. The role of the American Medical Association (AMA) in blocking national health insurance[4] and in shaping the Medicare-Medicaid legislation[5] has been well documented. There have also been several case studies of the AMA as a pressure group.[6] The pressure group behavior of physicians has also been studied in Britain,[7] Germany,[8] and Canada[9] and comparatively in Britain, the United States, and

Sweden.[10] The general lesson to emerge from these studies is that physicians as a group form a highly successful interest association, able to forge cohesive collective action, gain important concessions in the formation of public health programs, and block major features of health programs which are distasteful to them.

Although these studies have made a significant contribution to our understanding of the politics of the medical profession, the interest group approach misses a fundamental feature of professional power. Interest groups are generally defined as private associations, *outside* the government, which use their influence and power to affect the decisions made by government. The medical profession indeed functions as an interest group, but the profession itself is also a quasi-government with various kinds of de jure and de facto authority to govern the behavior of individual physicians, medical schools, and hospitals.

In the United States, the states have delegated considerable authority to the state boards of medical examiners, which are in turn generally controlled by the state medical societies. The boards of examiners have authority to issue and revoke licenses for the practice of medicine, a power which many observers have noted gives the profession the ability to restrict the supply of physicians.[11] The AMA also serves as an accrediting body (through its Council on Medical Education), and because all state boards of examiners require graduation from an approved medical school as a prerequisite for licensing, accreditation by the AMA is of vital importance to the medical schools. Through its accreditation procedures and powers, the AMA thus gains a strong influence over the nature of medical school curricula and the ability of medical schools to expand their class size. As postgraduate clinical training in hospital-run internship and residency programs has increased in prevalence and importance, the AMA has also been able to exert its influence on hospital policies.[12] Finally, the AMA and state medical societies have influenced the development of voluntary health insurance plans, both by successfully pushing through state laws restricting the types of insurance plans that may operate and by more informal tactics such as disciplinary measures against physicians participating in disapproved plans.[13]

In addition to this collective dimension of their power, physicians exercise considerable power through their individual decisions. Most importantly, they determine the volume and nature of medical services provided. Each physician makes numerous decisions about whether to participate in public programs (e.g., to provide care to Medicaid or Medicare patients, to participate in vaccination programs), whether to use particular drugs, techniques, and equipment in his practice, and whether to use particular medical interventions in each particular case. The aggregated therapeutic decisions of individual physicians form the pattern of care that is provided over the entire community.

Through their influence over the volume and nature of medical services, physicians have a significant effect on the cost of health services. Health economists have long noted that the health care market differs from a normal market for consumer goods in that the physician is not only the supplier of services but also the advisor to the patient/consumer in determining which medical goods should be purchased.[14] In addition, the pricing behavior of physicians directly affects the costs of both publicly and privately provided health services.[15]

Furthermore, while physicians have always been decision-makers in the sense of choosing diagnoses and therapies, under systems of third-party payment (i.e., either private or public health insurance programs), physicians serve in effect as proxy decisionmakers for the third-party payors. Where insurance programs agree to reimburse providers for whatever services a physician deems necessary, the physician is essentially making a purchasing decision for the payors (as well as a consumption decision for the patient). When the payor is the government, physicians are in the position of having spending authority for the government. In the case of Medicare and Medicaid, payment is open-ended; rather than a fixed sum of money's being allocated by Congress for the purpose of health services to the eligible beneficiaries, payment is made on a fee-for-service basis for any services which a physician deems necessary.

Finally, physicians as individuals wield a great deal of power through their role as gatekeepers for a variety of nonmedical benefits and privileges that are somehow contingent on certification of medical illness. Talcott Parsons, in a classic essay on social roles of patients and physicians,[16] noted that one important feature of illness as a social role is that the sick person typically is not held responsible for his condition and is exempted from normal social obligations. When the exemptions apply to civic duties or contractual obligations, rather than simply to personal obligations within personal relationships, physicians are often used as agents of the state or organization granting the exemption to certify the legitimacy of claims. Thus, for example, physicians are used to certify illness for people wishing to be exempt from military drafts, from jury duty, or from testifying when subpoenaed. In the Soviet Union, where labor is an obligation to the state and unjustified absence is a crime, workers must have a sick leave certificate signed by a physician in order to avoid penalty.[17] In countries where health insurance programs also include wage continuation payments during illness, such as England and Germany, a sick leave certificate from a physician is necessary in order to collect the cash benefits. Physicians, then, are often in the position of making discretionary decisions that determine the allocation of benefits and privileges among individual citizens.

Physicians, then, exercise political power both collectively and individually. Collectively, they function as a strong legislative and bureaucratic pressure group, able to influence legislation and administrative regulations concerning health care. In addition, the medical profession, through its associations, often serves as an agency of government for areas of policymaking and implementation for which it has been delegated authority by the state. Individually, physicians make discretionary decisions that determine the volume and nature of medical services, the cost of medical services, and the allocation of many nonmedical benefits associated with illness.

The Sources of Physicians' Power

Social scientists are only beginning to explore the sources of physicians' power. One major question in the study of the politics of medical care is the extent to which professional power derives from the nature of medical care itself or, alternatively, the extent to which professional power is shaped and limited by the political context in which it operates. If the power of physicians is primarily due to some inherent characteristics of medicine, such as complexity, or salience to a wide spectrum of citizens, then governments are indeed constrained in the kinds of public health policy decisions they can make. Major changes in government health policy, in the organization and delivery of services, or in the allocation of resources within the health sector and between health and other sectors will require major changes in the social and technical character of medicine. If, on the other hand, the power of the medical profession derives from the allocation of authority and the nature of decision-making structures within a particular political system, governments may have more scope for the reorientation of public policy in health care. The implications of this theory of professional power are that governments can increase their power vis-à-vis doctors by altering the organizational framework and the structure of incentives within which doctors work.

Comparative studies of medical care politics provide a useful way to approach this problem of identifying the sources of physicians' power. If professional power is indeed primarily a function of the nature of health services, we should expect to find very few differences in the political strength of medical professions among various advanced nations where the technology of medicine is relatively similar. If physicians' power derives primarily from the institutionalized patterns of decision-making about health policy in a given country, then we might expect to see conflicts between doctors and governments that focus on these institutional factors, and we might expect to see victories by either party.

The comparative study of health care politics is not yet advanced enough to permit the resolution of this question. The field is still at the stage of providing case studies of national health care systems. But the question has at least been raised: To what extent is behavior shaped by national political contexts, and to what extent are there inherent characteristics of the medical profession as such which override national differences and result in overwhelming similarities across nations in the resolution of public policy conflicts in the field of health care? This issue is most fully discussed in some of the work of Harry Eckstein[18] and of Theodore Marmor and David Thomas.[19]

Harry Eckstein, in a classic study of the British Medical Association, argues that specific political and social factors of a nation determine the nature and effectiveness of the activities of pressure groups in the system. Eckstein is concerned with explaining three dimensions of pressure group behavior, namely, the channels of influence developed and used by the group, the scope and intensity of pressure group activity, and the effectiveness of pressure group activity. In a theoretical chapter preceding the case study of the British Medical Association, he suggests that there are three major determinants of pressure group activities, all having to do with the characteristics of the political system within which pressure groups operate. These factors are the structure of government (e.g., the locus and concentration of power in the sphere of interest of the pressure group); the activities and policies of the government (e.g., whether the government pursues positive programs that require detailed administration, and whether the government engages in regulating the activities of the pressure group); and finally, attitudes, both about politics in general and about the issues of concern to the pressure group (e.g., cultural norms about legitimate political tactics and about the importance of medical care).

Marmor and Thomas dispute Eckstein's generalizations and argue instead that physicians have such enormous political and economic resources by virtue of the nature of the services they produce that national political contexts are comparatively insignificant as determinants of professional influence, at least for certain kinds of medical policy decisions. They offer the following hypothesis:

> Whatever the political and medical structure of a western industrialized country, physician preferences determine the governmental methods of payment. . . . As producers of a crucial service in industrial countries, and a service for which governments can seldom provide short-run substitutions, physicians have overwhelming political resources to influence decisions regarding payment methods quite apart from the form of bargaining their organizations employ.[20]

Their explanation is based on a set of assumptions about the preferences and behavior of doctors and government. The essential assumptions are: doctors prefer the payment methods that prevailed before the introduction of public programs; government officials perceive doctors as willing to strike over issues of payment method; and government officials are not willing to risk such a strike.

Marmor and Thomas place several limitations on their hypothesis. First, their arguments are limited to "western industrial countries." Second, they state that their hypothesis holds when two conditions are met: "when intense and widespread doctors' preferences are known by the actors in the decision-making process, and when large additional public funding is not entailed."[21] The hypothesis is thus actually very narrow; it covers only a certain kind of policy issue (payment methods), and within that issue, applies only to incremental changes. By excluding situations where "large additional public funding is entailed," the authors exclude all those situations where governments embark on major new public programs.

Given the reasoning behind the hypothesis—namely, that physicians' power derives from the crucial nature of the services they produce—one is led to ask whether the hypothesis can be extended. If the services of physicians are indeed crucial and irreplaceable, physicians' political power should extend to a range of situations, including major policy disputes and issues other than payment levels and methods. And although Marmor and Thomas do not try to extend their arguments beyond the specific question they examine, their reasoning raises the serious question of whether the nature of medical care and of people's attitudes toward health care renders physicians a special international elite.

Two basic arguments have been advanced by scholars to support the notion that the power of physicians is primarily due to some inherent characteristics of medicine as a field. One argument is that the high degree of technical expertise required both to practice medicine and to understand or evaluate medical care is at the core of the profession's power.[22] The complex technology used in the practice of medicine and the sophisticated basic science knowledge necessary to understand physiological processes are features that are thought to require a dependence of lay persons on the medical profession in all questions having to do with health and illness. But technical expertise alone certainly cannot account for the great power of the medical profession. Many areas of modern life require substantial technical expertise, yet many groups possessing such expertise are not nearly so powerful as physicians. One has only to think of engineers, research scientists, or computer programmers to find some counterexamples.

Many scholars have advanced versions of another argument, namely, that there is a distinct set of cultural ideas and values about health and medical care that provides a strong ideological rationale for the political autonomy of the medical profession.[23] There are several elements to this rationale. First is the paradigm of illness that is prevalent in Western society, in which disease is thought to be caused by some external agent that "invades" the body.[24] The germ theory of disease is by now a popular as well as a professional conception. The importance of this paradigm is that it entails a belief that disease requires some kind of human intervention in turn, in order to fight off the cause of the disease; thus physicians become the "heroes" capable of fighting the invaders. Many writers have pointed out the interventionist bias of physicians in clinical practice and of the health care system in general.[25] The basic paradigm of illness thus leads to a generalized belief in the ability of physicians to provide good health, or at least to mitigate the consequences of illness.

A second element of the ideological rationale for the autonomy of the medical profession is the high value people put on good health and physical well-being. Doctors are accorded a high degree of respect and autonomy because they provide a service that is highly valued. Parsons emphasizes that in the American value system, health is valued not only for its own sake, but also because good health is a prerequisite to other kinds of achievements that are highly valued.[26] Other research indicates that health is valued differently by different social groups within the United States,[27] and that many people engage in risky or dangerous behavior that would seem to indicate a low value on longevity and good health.[28] Nonetheless, the notion that good health is an important value to most people persists as an explanation for the strong power of physicians relative to other kinds of technical experts.

A third element of the ideological rationale is the concept of the doctor-patient relationship. Physicians have claimed that a warm personal relationship based on a strong sense of trust in the physician by the patient is *therapeutically* necessary to effective medical care. The therapeutic function of this relationship is then used to justify the profession's claim to autonomy and resistance to any kind of government intervention in the practice of medicine, including government involvement in the financing of health services.[29]

Finally, many people have argued that there is a tendency in Western societies to treat more and more forms of deviance as illnesses.[30] Thomas Szasz describes how judgments that are really moral condemnations are written as if they were medical diagnoses.[31] Sociologists of crime have increasingly interpreted criminal behavior as symptoms of individual pathology, and most efforts at reforming the criminal justice system in the recent past have been predicated on notions of treatment rather than punishment.[32] In the most sweeping critique of the "medicalization" of modern society, Ivan Illich argues that the paradigm of individual pathology as the cause of many problems, such as malnutrition, automobile accidents, and poor health, diverts popular attention and political action away from aspects of social organization and political power that cause and perpetuate these social problems.[33] The common thread in all these points of view is that the increased importance of the concept of illness in many areas of social life is thought to explain increases in physicians' political power.

The Limits of Physicians' Power

One of the central issues of democratic theory is how a government can be structured so as to control the use of political power by very strong groups. Three concepts in particular have been dominant in American thinking about mechanisms to achieve political accountability. These are representative democracy, pluralism, and free market competition. For various reasons, none of these mechanisms is appropriate to the kind of political power exercised by the medical profession, and, as we will see, rather different types of control mechanisms have been created in the sphere of medicine.

The notion of representative democracy implies that policy is made ultimately by elected representatives of the population at large. People's policy preferences are (in theory) translated into votes, which in turn put into office representatives who formulate and enact programs consistent with the will of their constituents. Accountability is built into the system through the frequency of elections; representatives are elected for some limited time period, after which they must resubmit themselves to the public, or step down altogether. The necessity to go before the public in periodic elections keeps representatives somewhat responsive to the needs and demands of the general citizenry.

Clearly, representative democracy is hardly applicable to physicians. The most important reason is that long training is required to gain the expertise necessary to practice medicine, so that periodic elections of new physicians would not make much sense.[34] In practice, although physicians are often in the position of exercising governmental authority, they are in no way representative of any kind of popular will. Physicians are not chosen in any kind of public process; rather, they are self-selected into a pool of applicants to medical schools, and then chosen by the medical schools which are themselves usually private organizations.

Another central notion in American democratic theory is pluralism. In a pluralistic system, citizens form and join groups to represent their particular interests, and policy is derived through the interaction of these groups in the political arena. Controls on excess power are achieved in two ways. First, each citizen has multiple interests and is likely to belong to many diverse groups. The groups thus have overlapping memberships, and no one group can become overwhelmingly large. Second, there are many different politically active groups within the society, and the competition among these groups serves as a check on the power of any one group.[35]

Regardless both of how one assesses the accuracy of this interpretation of American politics and of how one evaluates the efficacy of pluralism as a mechanism for political accountability, it is easy to see that the idea is not easily applicable to the medical profession. On a theoretical level, there is fundamental incompatibility between the notion of expertise and the notion of competition. Expertise implies that there are right and wrong ways (or more and less effective ways) of achieving some outcome or solving some problem, and that a choice of means should be based on correctness. The pluralist notion of competition among groups rests on an assumption that the choices to be made are among *preferences* and *opinions*, not among right or wrong answers. One goal of any health care system is certainly to optimize the utilization of expert knowledge. Although it may be argued that competition among different schools of thought and methods of practice is useful to spur innovation and to generate new knowledge, clearly some limits to diversity are called for when enough knowledge is gained to demonstrate the clear superiority of one school or method.

The practical limits of pluralism as a controlling device in the field of medical care are equally serious. Although the medical profession is not a homogeneous group with no internal conflicts, the field of health care could hardly be characterized as one in which there is serious competition by rival groups for control over significant resources and policies. The medical profession has a legalized monopoly not only over the right to practice medicine, but also over entry into the profession, the training of physicians, and many aspects of the organization of health services.[36]

Pluralism is very much akin to the economists' notion of free market competition. Several theorists have interpreted group politics as a market in which political organizations compete for members by providing political or economic benefits.[37] In the perfectly competitive free market, competition for buyers among different sellers who produce inefficiently or who provide inferior quality goods will either change sellers' behavior or force them out of the market altogether. Ideally, the operation of a free market yields a socially optimum production and distribution of goods and allows for the satisfaction of minority tastes in a way that majority rule democracy cannot.

In the case of medical care, pure market competition cannot be counted as an effective regulatory device, again both for theoretical and for practical reasons.[38] The most important argument against consumer control in the medical field is that patients lack the knowledge to evaluate different providers of services and different choices presented to them by a single provider. Although the inability of lay persons to evaluate medical information is probably overestimated (both by the general population and by the medical profession), there are clearly many kinds of choices for which patients and politicians would want to rely on experts. The crucial political problem is to design a system that utilizes expert knowledge where appropriate but does not allow the political power of physicians to expand beyond the areas in which their expertise is genuine and relevant.[39]

There are also some very practical reasons why market competition does not work in the health care field. Because of restrictions on advertising imposed by the medical profession on itself, consumers lack access to practical information necessary for informed choice. It is difficult for a patient to find out about office hours, experience of a physician in treating particular problems, or fees. Another obstacle to real competition among physicians is that they are in short supply in many geographical areas and in many subareas of medicine, so that consumers do not face a real choice among providers.

Representative democracy, pluralism, and free market competition are generally thought to be inappropriate types of controls for the medical profession and, in fact, the controls imposed on physicians are of a different sort. The most striking feature of existing political structures for ensuring accountability of physicians is that they are concerned almost exclusively with standards of clinical performance rather than with the collective or individual power of physicians in a political sense. There are three major control mechanisms by which the behavior of physicians is regulated in the current practice of American medicine.[40] These mechanisms are informal peer review, formal self-regulation, and tort law.

From the point of view of the medical profession, informal peer review is the most congruent with professional norms. Since the medical profession holds that only other physicians are qualified to judge a physician's work, it puts a large emphasis on the sufficiency of internal review mechanisms and the destructiveness of outside control. Peer review, in theory, means that physicians control the quality of their performance by informally observing each other's work and offering suggestions and criticisms where appropriate.

In practice, peer review does not apparently work very much like the theory. Peer review as a control mechanism has three essential components, each of which must function in order for peer review to work. First, physicians must be able to observe each other's work. Second, physicians must be willing to criticize each other when they disagree over techniques, diagnoses, and standards of therapy. And finally, physicians must have and be willing to exercise sanctions. Current research suggests that these conditions are rarely met.[41] Freidson has demonstrated that the visibility of physicians' work is associated with the relation of various specialties in the division of labor. To the extent that physicians do observe each other's work, it is through referral networks: physicians treating the same patient may have some idea of each other's quality of performance.[42] But the logic of referral networks means that visibility will be higher *across* specialties, since referral is usually made to a physician in a different specialty. Thus, the physicians least competent to evaluate the performance of any given specialist are the ones most likely to have information about it. Other than the sharing of patients, there is no mechanism by which physicians systematically (or even sporadically) observe each other's work.

Peer review also seems to falter on the willingness of physicians to criticize each other and to use available sanctions. Freidson found that "talking to" a peer was the only institutionalized punishment used by physicians short of dismissal, and dismissal was distinctly a last resort for egregious cases.[43] Physicians may cease referring patients to another physician whose work they deem inferior. Although such an informal boycott is an available sanction, its use is antithetical to the improvement of care. Ceasing referral does not communicate any constructive information to the offending physician and only creates isolated networks of physicians with similar standards of practice.[44]

In addition to informal peer review, the medical profession is somewhat controlled by more formal methods of self-regulation. Medical discipline is carried out by two different types of physicians' organizations: medical societies, which are private professional associations, and state boards of medical examiners, which are quasi-governmental organizations.

Medical societies, as professional associations, have typically been more concerned with advancing the art and knowledge of medicine (through seminars, symposia, continuing education programs) and with trade union issues (income of physicians, methods of payment, minimizing competition among physicians) than with monitoring the clinical competence of their members. A 1964 survey of all state medical societies (47 of 51 responded) found that only eight had some provision in their constitution or bylaws allowing disciplinary action to be taken against an incompetent physician.[45] In each of these eight states, the only action that could be taken against an incompetent physician was removal from membership. Since a medical society is only a professional association, exclusion from membership does not prevent a physician from continuing to practice. The lack of any formal provision for monitoring physician competence by the overwhelming majority of state medical societies indicates that these bodies do not see themselves as watchdogs of clinical performance.

State boards of medical examiners are administrative agencies of state governments. Each state, through its medical practice act, delegates authority to the board to license physicians for practice within the state and to discipline physicians for certain offenses (defined with varying degrees of specificity in the different state acts). Although the state boards are probably the most important mechanism for the regulation of physicians' behavior, their regulatory powers are severely hampered by political, economic, and legal constraints.

Most states require that boards be composed entirely of licensed practicing physicians. Some states use one board, composed of a variety of health professionals, to license all the health occupations. In practice, the state boards are often closely related to the state medical societies. In twenty-three states the state medical society has some direct authority in the appointment of the boards; sixteen states *require* that the governor choose board members from a list of candidates submitted by the medical society, and several other states follow that procedure. In two states (North Carolina and Maryland), members are selected directly by the medical associations.[46] Thus, in many cases the procedure for appointing the state boards of examiners ensures that they are controlled by the state medical societies.[47]

As agencies of the state, the boards of medical examiners are usually dependent on the state budgeting process for the allocation of their funds.[48] Low funding, and the consequent lack of an investigatory staff, are considered severe problems for the boards. In addition, the boards often lack the legal expertise (or funds to acquire it) necessary for them to engage in aggressive regulation of the profession, since any disciplinary action against a physician almost always entails an administrative hearing with stringent legal standards.

The disciplinary function of state boards is also limited by the nature of their legal authority. They are administrative bodies which have the power to enforce the laws of the state. Thus, they may discipline physicians only for offenses specified by the medical practice acts of their respective states. There is great variety among the different laws, but the most comonly included offenses for which a board can revoke or suspend the license of a physician are: illegal abortion (prior to the Supreme Court decision of 1972 legalizing first-trimester abortions); certain kinds of advertising; conviction of a crime or felony; fraud in obtaining a license; narcotics violations; sexual misbehavior; and moral turpitude.[49] As can be seen from this list, the disciplinary authority of boards is focused on abuses of the state's own laws (often ones which have nothing to do with medical care per se). The boards do not often have the legal authority to monitor the clinical performance of physicians.

In some states, the medical practice act includes a more general offense, such as "unprofessional conduct," "manifest incapacity," or "gross carelessness," which can be used by the boards to discipline specifically technical incompetence, as opposed to violations of criminal laws. The courts of different states have handed down different opinions as to whether such phrases as "unprofessional conduct" are sufficiently precise as to provide a clear standard of behavior; some courts have held that such phrases are too vague and in effect delegate legislative authority to the boards of examiners.[50] Hence, the ability of state boards of medical examiners to discipline physicians for technical incompetence may be limited by their legislative authority.

In practice, the disciplinary action of state boards has been quite limited. A survey by the Federation of State Medical Boards found that between 1964 and 1974 there were 1,978 disciplinary actions by state boards, of which approximately forty-eight percent involved narcotics abuse.[51] The work of the boards is indeed concentrated on violations of criminal law mostly unrelated to the practice of medicine (except insofar as narcotics addiction may be deemed to render one incapable of practicing medicine), and they rarely use their power to discipline for incompetence under the generic offenses "unprofessional conduct" and "gross malpractice".

The judicial system provides a mechanism through which physicians may be held directly accountable for damages they cause. Patients may sue their physicians for bad medical outcomes resulting from substandard care. The traditional standard used to judge physician performance is one of "customary practice," meaning that each physician is normally held accountable only to the practices and procedures used by his peers within the profession, rather than to any outside evaluation or standard of judgment.[52] The customary practice standard has in the past been interpreted to mean that there might be different standards in different communities, depending on the usual patterns of practice, though some courts have recently moved toward enforcing a national standard of care.[53] Because malpractice law relies on the doctrine of customary practice, malpractice becomes in effect a mode of enforcing peer standards; although the sanctions may be more harsh than those of internal peer review mechanisms, the standards are probably no more stringent.

In theory, the medical malpractice system disciplines substandard physicians by making them compensate for negligent care, and protects society by deterring others from the same or similar conduct and perhaps also by putting low quality physicians at a competitive disadvantage. In practice, there are several reasons why civil liability does not provide an adequate mechanism through which physicians may be held accountable to the public. First, only some of the patients who are harmed by deficient medical practices are inclined and financially able to bring claims against their physicians. Second, the system of tort liability provides at best primarily after-the-fact compensation. The deterrence effect is mitigated by physician liability insurance, since most malpractice claims are paid by insurance companies and not by physicians themselves. And because liability insurance premiums are based on the malpractice experience of categories of physicians rather than on each individual physician's experience,[54] the fees charged by individual physicians do not truly reflect their differential malpractice experience, or allow the consumer to differentiate among them. Also, physicians tend to perceive the outcomes of malpractice claims as random events shaped by the vagaries of bad medical outcomes, patient litigiousness, out-of-court bargaining procedures, and the whims of particular juries, so that their perception of the malpractice system may not lead them to alter their professional practice in any way.[55]

A third reason for the inadequacy of tort liability is that fear of malpractice suits may lead physicians to practice "defensive medicine," in which they perform unnecessary diagnostic tests and therapeutic procedures or refuse to undertake particularly risky courses of treatment in order to protect themselves from later suits. In various surveys, substantial proportions of physicians have claimed that they practice defensive medicine, but attempts to measure the extent of defensive medical practice have been inconclusive so far.[56]

Finally, the current crisis in malpractice insurance[57] demonstrates that the system is not viable when large numbers of patients actually assert their rights and make claims against physicians. Physicians themselves are finding the cost of premiums unacceptably high, and insurance companies are finding malpractice insurance so costly that they are ceasing to carry it.

These traditional mechanisms of physician accountability—peer review, self-regulation, and tort law—would be inadequate controls over the political authority of physicians, even if they functioned well. None of these mechanisms is designed to monitor or check the power asserted by the medical profession collectively, either as a pressure group or as an association with delegated authority of the state. And even though these mechanisms are designed to deal with the competence of individual physicians, they are not concerned with the impact of physicians' discretionary decisions on public policy.

To the extent that broader controls over the power of the medical profession have been a subject of the American public policy debate, American solutions have typically been based on the idea of structuring authority so as to *fragment* strong groups. The notion that power can best be contained by fragmenting strong interests into smaller groups that compete with each other is a fundamental tenet of American political theory, most explicitly expressed in Madison's Tenth Federalist Paper. Most of the proposals for redesign of the American health system that have emerged in recent years are variants on the theme of fragmenting the power of the medical profession. One current of reform would have the government foster marketlike competition, in which different "providers" of health services would be held in check by competition with each other, and the "public interest" would emerge through the assertion of "consumer preferences." Government's role would be to bolster the purchasing strength of consumers, by providing health insurance, tax credits, or vouchers, for example. In another variation on the fragmentation theme, government's role would be to foster the development of multiple health service providers offering alternative services, such as health maintenance organizations. In still another variant, the government would fragment the medical profession by vigorously applying antitrust policy, to eliminate the anticompetitive rules and practices.

The German political system has taken an entirely different approach to the problem of controlling physicians' professional power. Instead of fragmenting the medical profession to keep it weak, the government deliberately *consolidated* it, but confronted it with strong countervailing organizations. Physicians are concentrated into a few large political organizations, required to negotiate as a collective unit, and forced to fight among themselves for the limited social resources devoted to medical care. The government takes a similar role with other social interests, including the interests of health service users. Government created and fosters the development of large organizations of insured persons that can bargain on an equal footing with physicians.

This book, is a case study of an alternate system for controlling the power of the medical profession. Although medicine in West Germany is characterized by the same kinds of technical expertise and by very similar cultural values and ideas as we have described for the United States, the relationship between the medical profession and the state is quite different. Several structural features of German politics will be examined in order to demonstrate that much of the political power of physicians can be accounted for by characteristics of the political system and by political decisions, rather than by the technical nature of medical care or by ideological beliefs and values about health care. The West German national health insurance system grows out of a political tradition very different from our own, yet the contrast is highly illuminating.

The Corporatist Context of Physician Politics | Chapter Two

The Original National Health Insurance Scheme

Public health insurance in Germany began in the late nineteenth century as part of a conservative social policy whose main aim was to preserve the old social order. The current system of health insurance and the political relationships it entails can best be understood with reference to the ideological and political struggles that shaped them. Even today, West German social policy is based on principles that are fundamentally different from the liberal assumptions underlying American social policy.

When a public health insurance program was introduced by Chancellor Bismarck's government in 1883, Germany had only recently become a unified nation-state, after defeating France in 1870. It was far less advanced on the road to economic modernization than either France or England. Historians have attributed much to the fact of Germany's late industrialization and the country's alleged desire to "catch up" with stronger economic powers of Western Europe. Regardless of how one assesses the importance of timing in German economic development, it is clear that the *pattern* of industrialization in Germany had important consequences for the development of political and social institutions.

The central political problem of Bismarck's government was how to industrialize the country without disturbing the existing political order. Conservatives envisioned society as an organic entity, and used the image of the social "fabric" to represent the notion that the various parts of society were interwoven and interdependent, so that a disruption of any part might lead to a disintegration of the whole. In Conservative ideology, political and economic conflict could best be contained by corporative organization.[1] Corporatism, as the term will be used here, is a mode of political organization with two particular characteristics. First, the intermediary between the citizen and the government is a compulsory membership organization (or set of organizations) based primarily on occupational status. And second, these organizations are granted statutory authority to control work-related aspects of their members' behavior and to administer government programs related to the members.

For the Conservatives, the handicraft guilds of skilled artisans epitomized the ideal combination of economic productivity and stable, hierarchical political authority. The guild system of production was for the Conservatives what the factory system was for the Liberals. The factory system required a redefinition of political and social relationships such that individual workers would be free to move from place to place and sell their labor to the highest bidder. Obligations between employer and employee would be purely contractual, based only on formal agreement between the individual parties involved and not on social class or other characteristics. In contrast, the guild system required that producers belong to corporative trade associations which had authority to regulate all practices connected with the particular trades, and which advised the government and represented the interests of the trade to the government. Within each guild, occupational relationships were clearly defined, and exact requirements for training of apprentices and certification of masters were specified and administered. Each trade had its own occupational court to arbitrate conflicts among parties within that trade. Even methods of production and selling were closely regulated by the guilds. The notion that political interests can best be represented by a set of stable, occupationally based membership groups is a profound tradition in German politics which has significantly influenced the structure of social welfare programs.

The Conservative answer to the problem of combining industrial development with the political status quo was to foster "reform from above." If the state were the sponsor of industrialization, it could better control not only the pace but also the mode of development. The most important feature of the German pattern of industrialization was that the state was simultaneously the protector of old social elites and the guarantor of new economic development. On the one hand, the state adopted economic and legal policies to protect the old landed aristocracy. Tariffs on imported grains were both materially and symbolically important as a policy that protected the large Prussian estates against competition from more efficient foreign farmers and allowed traditional patterns of ownership and political relationships of the countryside to remain intact.[2] On the other hand, the state was also "the largest single entrepreneur"[3] in Germany's industrial development. The state provided substantial capital in the form of interest-free loans to nascent German industries, as well as substantial support in the form of protectionist tariffs. In addition, the state was a major provider of administrative talent, in that the government either owned numerous enterprises (e.g., railroads, canals, mines, utilities) or participated in mixed public-private ventures.[4]

Bismarck's protectionist policies extended beyond the landed aristocracy and the new industrialists to include the emerging class of urban laborers. In fact, one writer has called Bismarck's social policy the "counterpart for labor of the protection offered to German industry."[5] Perhaps the greatest fear of Bismarck's government was the Social Democratic Party would capture the loyalties of the urban proletariat and would be strong enough to overthrow the existing order. To avoid this possibility, Bismarck made a two-pronged attack on the Socialists. After a Conservative electoral victory in 1878, he simply outlawed the Social Democratic Party; the ban lasted until 1890. But this negative approach was not sufficient, as King William I said in his message to the Reichstag of November 17, 1881: "Even in February of this year We have had our conviction expressed that the healing of the social damages cannot be sought exclusively by way of the repression of Social Democratic riots, but will have to be sought equally in the positive promotion of the welfare of the workers."[6] And so the government passed a series of social welfare measures whose explicit aim was to solidify the workers' loyalty to the state. In 1883, 1884, and 1889, the government initiated social insurance programs for illness, accident, and old age, respectively. The goal of these programs was to buy political support from the workers in exchange for economic security and material benefits. As with Disraeli's social reforms in England in the mid–nineteenth century, Bismarck's state welfare measures arose from a conservative political impulse, however progressive the material benefits might be.[7]

Accident insurance was actually the first of the social welfare programs to be advocated and debated, and the tenor of the debate is very revealing of the conservative goals and intentions behind the entire social insurance scheme.[8] Because the purpose of social insurance was to bind the workers to the state, it was important to Bismarck that the insurance benefits not be financed entirely or even mostly by employers; the workers, he thought, should know that their welfare was paid for by the state. In the original accident insurance bill submitted in 1881, workers were to pay less than half of the premiums, on a graduated scale according to income. The remainder was to come from employer contributions and heavy state subsidy. The system was to be administered by a government insurance office. The state would retain control, and private insurance companies were to be excluded. Rimlinger points out that Bismarck was more concerned with the effect of social insurance programs on the workers' attitudes than on their welfare. "If the worker has to pay for it himself, the effect on him will be lost," Bismarck jotted on a report.[9]

The first accident insurance bill met with overwhelming opposition in the Reichstag, and two more bills were debated before one finally passed in 1884. Bismarck's second line of defense had been a system of corporative organizations that would provide a link between individuals and a central office; he foresaw this system of corporative representation as another institution of popular representation that would share legislative authority with the Reichstag. Needless to say, the Reichstag members were heavily opposed to this proposal. The elected representatives were not anxious to eliminate their own role in government, either by tying workers directly to a central office of the state or by integrating them into alternate intermediary organizations.

Ultimately, the bill that passed provided for decentralized administration of accident insurance by employers' associations, with employers paying almost the full cost of the scheme. Bismarck failed to achieve either financial dependence of the worker on the state or political integration of workers through corporative organizations with administrative responsibility for the social insurance.

The national health insurance program was politically more successful. Bismarck again failed to achieve his goal of administering the program through state insurance offices—this time partly because of resistance by existing mutual aid societies that provided health insurance. The first compulsory health insurance program grafted a new scheme onto the preexisting system of private insurance, organized and marketed through work groups. But Bismarck's government *was* able to create a series of corporative associations to administer national health insurance. These "sickness funds" (*Krankenkassen*) were jointly managed by workers and their employers and were given exclusive authority to administer the national health insurance program. The existing mutual aid societies were called "substitute funds" and allowed to handle insurance for the national program. The health insurance program was thus a political success in two senses. It tied the worker's social benefits directly to his employer (and less directly to the state), thus providing some disincentive for higher wage demands and for searching out new employment. And it made the sickness funds joint organizations of employers and employees, which undermined any future effort of trade unions to capture social protection as an exclusive function of labor organizations.

The first health insurance program already had several essential elements of the current system. First, there was compulsory membership in a sickness fund for a defined group of workers, those with the occupational title *Arbeiter* ("blue-collar worker") or earning under RM 2,000. It is important to note that people were included in the compulsory health insurance scheme by virtue of their *occupational position*, rather than their need for health care. One might argue, as some politicians did, that need was in fact a criterion for inclusion, since the earnings figure used to determine membership was a measure of financial need. But since the earnings criterion was not applied to all people—not to tradesmen, craftsmen, the self-employed, farmers, the unemployed, or family members of working people—it is clear that even financial need was not the major criterion. To be eligible for compulsory health insurance, one had to be a manual worker. In the current system, eligibility has been expanded to almost all occupational groups, but occupation is still the major determinant of eligibility for the different types of funds.

A second principle of the current system that could be seen in the original system was the administration of the health insurance program through numerous small, independent sickness funds with statutory authority to manage the program. The protection of social interests through compulsory membership societies is quite similar to the corporatist idea of protection of economic and political interests through compulsory guilds.

Third, the original program already included the provision that the broad outlines of the scheme—the criteria for defining the population to be covered, the level of contributions to the scheme, and the types of cash and service benefits to be provided by the funds—were all to be determined by the legislature (the Reichstag).

Fourth, from the very beginning the system was financed by contributions from employers and employees. Originally employees paid two-thirds and employers one-third of the costs; this proportion has been changed to half-and-half, but the basic principle of financing through employer-employee contributions, rather than by state subsidies from general revenues, remains an essential ingredient of the system.

Finally, the national health insurance system always included a measure of self-management, i.e., participation by the contributors to the scheme in the management of the sickness funds. Employers and employees were granted representation on the governing bodies of the individual funds in proportion to their contributions; thus, workers originally held two-thirds of the seats on self-management committees. The principle of self-management by the contributors served both to answer the Liberal demands for more democratic participation, and to contain industrial conflict by pitting workers and employers against each other in a controlled setting.

Employer and employee representation in sickness fund management was another reflection of the corporatist principle that political interests are best represented through occupational groupings. Conservatives generally favored voting systems based on group representation. On the question of a national electoral system, they wanted the franchise to be based on occupational and social class categories, rather than on property ownership or on universal manhood suffrage. Under such a system, each particular occupational category (such as large estate owners, managers of medium estates, day laborers, and so on) would elect representatives to a national legislature. The number of representatives would be weighted both by the proportion of the total population in each occupational group and by the social importance of each group.[10] The system of representation within the sickness funds was a clear victory of Conservative principles. Individuals were represented not as such, but as members of a group with a particular relationship to the system of production. This attachment of the right of representation to the level of financial contributions led to a curious twist in party politics: the Social Democrats found themselves supporting high contributions by workers (i.e., a high proportion of the cost), so that workers would gain the political power attached to contributions by the design of the program.[11]

The Contemporary National Health Insurance Scheme

The contemporary health insurance scheme can be understood only with reference to the principles of the original scheme. The system is based on laws made at the federal level and codified into what is still known as the Imperial Insurance Code (Reichsversicherungsordnung). As the program expanded, the new laws were constantly added on to the old, with no recodification. The code known as the "RVO," can be found on the desk of virtually every administrator in the health care field. In 1975, the government finally undertook to consolidate the social insurance regulations, but the new version (the Sozialgesetzbuch) will take several years to complete.

The federal law defines important outlines of the system. It stipulates the population to be covered under compulsory insurance, by defining the occupational categories for which insurance is compulsory. The law also stipulates the amount of contributions to the scheme (and thus also influences the total amount of money available for health care) by specifying the wage base subject to taxation (*Grundlohn*). (As in the American Social Security system, only a limited portion of a worker's income is taxed; the ceiling on taxable earnings is set by the legislature.) In 1951, the share of employees' contributions was reduced from two-thirds to one-half, and the employers' share was correspondingly increased from one-third to one-half. Finally, federal laws also determine the basic benefits that must be offered by every sickness fund.

The citizen's relationship to the health insurance scheme is defined by position in the work force, as indicated by occupation and earnings. All blue-collar workers (i.e., manual workers) are required to participate in the public health insurance scheme, regardless of income. White-collar workers must participate if their earnings are below a level set by the federal government each year (*Versicherungspflichtgrenze*). In 1978, this level was DM 33,000 per year. The minimum income for exemption is considerably higher than the average income. In 1976, the exemption level was DM 27,900, and the mean income from wages and salaries was about DM 22,000. People earning higher amounts and the self-employed may participate voluntarily. The distinction between blue and white-collar jobs is based on whether the work is primarily physical or mental. The question of job classification, because it determines insurance obligations and benefits, has often been litigated in the social courts.[12]

Although membership in health insurance is defined by categories of work and earnings, people who do not or cannot work are also covered. This occurs in several ways. The contribution of any wage earner automatically covers all of his or her dependents. The tax rate and the wage base for contributions remain fixed, so that the worker who earns DM 1,500 per month and has a large family pays exactly the same premium as the single worker earning the same income. Unemployed persons continue membership in their former funds and have their premiums paid by the unemployment insurance authorities; pensioners have their premiums paid by the pension authorities.[13] Approximately 92 percent of the West German population belong to some version of the scheme and another 7 percent carry private or other health insurance, so that 99 percent of the population have some form of health insurance.[14] Of the people insured in the social insurance program, about 34 percent are compulsory members, 40 percent are dependents, 17 percent are pensioners, and 8 percent are voluntary members.[15]

Public health insurance is administered by about 1,400 sickness funds. Although the funds were originally organized around broad occupational categories (e.g., factory funds, guild funds, miner funds, mariner funds, student funds), now about half of the insured population belongs to local funds, which are residuals for people who do not come under the jurisdiction of the occupationally based funds.

All of the sickness funds are bodies of public law (*Körperschaften des öffentlichen Rechts*). This is a quasi-public status of German administrative law, in which interest group associations are granted statutory authority to administer public programs. The funds are authorized to set their premiums, collect the contributions from members and employers, and designate supplementary benefits beyond the federally mandated package. Technically, they can decide whether to authorize payment for each medical service, including a hospitalization, but in practice, the legislature and the courts have defined mandatory benefits quite precisely; the funds are authorized to monitor office-based services and withold payment for unnecessary ones, but they have little latitude to deny a hospitalization recommended by a physician.

The sickness funds are confronted by organizations of health care providers, with whom they contract for the care of their patients. In the ambulatory sector, they negotiate fee schedules with organizations of office-based physicians known as "associations of insurance doctors" (AIDs). In the hospital sector, a flat, per diem rate for each patient is officially set by an agency in each state (*Land*), but in practice is often the result of collective negotiation between the funds and the hospitals. Unlike the billing practices of American hospitals, whereby charges are levied separately for room and board, laboratory tests, use of other hospital facilities, and doctors' services, the daily charge of German hospitals covers room and board, nursing care, use of all facilities, *and* physicians' fees.

The AIDs, like the sickness funds, are bodies of public law. They are organized on a geographic basis, with local and state organizations and a national umbrella organization, the Federal Association of Insurance Doctors (*Kassenärztliche Bundesvereinigung*, or KBV). The AIDs are charged with ensuring that ambulatory health services are available to members of the public insurance system. In addition, whatever agreements an AID makes with sickness funds are binding on the individual physician members.

The sickness funds contract with the AIDs for ambulatory services to the fund members. In exchange for these services, each sickness fund pays the regional AID a quarterly sum of money, which is negotiated in advance and must cover the cost of services provided. Until the mid-1960s, the pool was generally established on a modified capitation basis, but after 1965, all of the funds gradually switched over to a fee-for-service method of setting the pool. The AID distributes this money to its members, using the fee schedule to allocate the pool. This payment system, then, is a two-stage process, combining a lump sum pool paid by the sickness funds to the AIDs with a fee-for-service distribution to individual physicians.

The German public health insurance system has preserved the private practice of medicine while subjecting physicians to fairly stringent and pervasive regulation. Unlike in the British and Swedish systems, most West German physicians are not direct government employees. And unlike in the American system, West German physicians do not have individual contracts with the public health insurance system, nor are their fees based on usual charges in private practice. National health insurance in West Germany presents an intermediate alternative between these two extremes.

The Health Insurance System in the Larger Context of Policymaking

The separation of patients and physicians into large-scale compulsory membership groups is the most important political feature of the West German national health insurance system. In the United States, health care is basically seen as an individual responsibility. Individuals are expected to fend for themselves in a free market, where they must seek out physicians, agree on prices, pay their own bills, and be responsible for their own budgets. Private health insurance is seen as an aid to individuals in carrying out these functions, and the role of public insurance is primarily to help people who are unable to obtain private insurance. In the West German system, there is no expectation that individuals should be able to obtain health care by themselves. The role of the sickness funds is to make physicians available, establish prices, handle all the financial transactions, and budget people's money for health care. All of these functions are performed by membership groups, which in turn enter into agreement with membership groups representing physicians. Neither physicians nor patients are expected or allowed to represent their own interests individually in the health care system.

This concentration of interests in the health sector into large compulsory membership groups is part of a profound tradition in German politics. The general characteristics that describe political organizations in the health sector are evident in other aspects of government, and it is important to understand that the methods used in West Germany for handling social policy problems are consistent with policymaking styles elsewhere in the government.

Analysts of West German policymaking structures have described the tendency to concentration in other sectors. Business ownership, and particularly bank ownership, tends to be much more concentrated than in the United States.[16] Anticartel and antitrust legislation is applied very weakly.[17] Germany has often been in a position of trying to industrialize or to recover economic productivity rapidly, and concentration of power in large firms has been a successful strategy.

Interest groups in the political system are similarly concentrated. Like Britain and Sweden, Germany has a series of "peak associations" or large, nationwide organizations that represent the political interests of various groups. Perhaps the three best-known examples are the Federation of German Employers' Unions (Bundesverband der deutschen Arbeitgeberverbände), the Federation of German Industry (Bundesverband der deutschen Industrie), and the German Association of Trade Unions (Deutscher Gewerkschaftsbund). The peak associations are unions of smaller groups, and they are assumed to speak in a single voice for their constituent member groups.

As in other parliamentary systems, most policymaking begins in the national bureaucracy. The vast majority of bills originate in the ministries—over eighty percent from 1949 to 1975[18]—and the tradition of strong party discipline, though not as strong as in Britain, means that bargaining over policy takes place mostly within the ministries during the process of legislative drafting.

Formal inclusion of interest groups in the policy formulation process is accomplished in two important ways. The ministries have the power to appoint special expert advisory commissions composed of representatives of the relevant interest groups and unaffiliated technical experts. The ministers are careful to balance the composition of the commissions to give fair representation to competing groups, and to counterbalance the explicitly partisan advice with that of independent experts. Commissions are an important source of technical information for the federal bureaucracy, and even more importantly, they are a source of political information about the needs, demands, and strengths of affected interest groups. The commissions are also a forum in which the organized interest groups bargain with each other, so that a consensus can be reached before the final bill is presented to the legislature.[19]

The ministries are also required to consult with the peak associations on major policy proposals, and they have developed a system of "bilateral contacts" with the interest groups to meet this requirement, especially where there are no established advisory commissions.[20] These contacts usually begin with a meeting of the heads of the interest group and a department or section head within the ministry. If conflicts cannot be resolved on this level, the issue is passed to successively higher levels, until some consensus is reached.[21] Since a program will usually not be submitted to Parliament unless there is consensus among all the cabinet departments, there is tremendous pressure on the individual departments to work out all the necessary compromises before the proposal is even submitted for cabinet approval. The policy process is not always so smooth in practice, however, as some major public controversies on health policy bills will attest.

The formal mechanisms for inclusion of interest groups in the process of policy implementation are equally well developed. Most important is the administrative device of the bodies of public law. These bodies are a hybrid between a private interest association and a public agency. Although they explicitly represent a set of identifiable economic and political interests, they are given two essential powers that interest associations do not have: statutory authority to make policy in their defined area of competence, and compulsory membership.

Occupational chambers are a type of body of public law, with authority to control the practices of a particular profession and to compel membership of all its practitioners. These chambers, which receive their authority from the *Länder* governments, grew out of the old guild traditions and have persisted as the mode of organizing and controlling professional conduct. For physicians, membership in the appropriate *Land*-level chamber is compulsory. The chambers are responsible for promulgating and enforcing a code of ethics, granting specialty certification, and generally handling matters of professional discipline. The *Land*-level chambers are organized into a voluntary national association, the Federal Chamber of Physicians (*Bundesärztekammer*, or BÄK), which, though lacking the status of a body of public law, is the peak association of physicians that is usually consulted on matters of health policy.

The quasi-public status granted to sickness funds, AIDs, and physician chambers obviously gives these groups (and other bodies of public law) significant power. When they engage in political controversies, they frequently emphasize that they represent public, not private, interests. Safran interprets this behavior as restraint: the public responsibilities of bodies of public law lead them to be "self-conscious and apologetic about exerting pressure."[22] The bodies of public law are in fact very active in political controversies that affect the material interests of their members, so it is not surprising that they attempt to build credibility by dissociating themselves from voluntary interest groups or by claiming to represent the "public interest."

In the American political system, there is no institution that is perfectly analogous to the bodies of public law. Some people would argue that regulatory agencies are often private interests in government clothing, and to the extent that a regulatory agency has been captured by its regulatees, it could be said to resemble a body of public law. But this situation is a long way from the German system, in which the blending of private interests and public authority is sanctioned in both political ideology and administrative law.

Regulation of professions is the one area of American political life where government policy comes closest to the corporatist model in Germany. For many professions, notably law and medicine, state governments have effectively delegated administrative authority to professional groups, in the form of state professional "boards." These boards have the authority to set educational and licensing standards, thereby controlling entry into the profession, and to set and enforce standards of practice. This resemblance between the two systems in their method of controlling professional groups makes the West German case all the more illuminating for the American scholar.

Although it is difficult to make any judgment about the relative power of American and West German physicians as legislative and bureaucratic pressure groups, analysis of their respective formal roles in the policymaking process suggests some important differences. West German physicians are represented by both private, independent, voluntary professional associations and quasi-governmental, compulsory membership organizations with responsibility for administration of government programs. The West German medical profession is more directly integrated into the structure of policymaking than the American and has access to more formal channels of influence. But because its institutionalized role derives from national patterns of political organization, its power may be counterbalanced by the similar roles and prerogatives accorded to its political adversaries.

Corporatist ideology permeates both the immediate context of physician politics—the national health insurance system—and the broader context of German politics in general. Underlying the social insurance system is a fundamental value placed on political stability and a belief that stability can be achieved by cementing individual loyalties to social groups within society, and by using a program of economic benefits to give the working class a material stake in the existing political system.[23] In the administrative structure of health insurance, and in the larger political system, political conflict is contained by the judicious grouping of individuals into compulsory membership organizations and the attachment of certain rights to these large groups rather than to the individual members The corporatist tradition helps to explain some of the sources of physicians' power that do not derive purely from technical expertise, and some of the mechanisms that German society has used to contain that power.

The concentration of competing interests in the health sector into large groups with statutory authority to administer the national health insurance program developed gradually over a period of at least fifty years. The system represents a particular way that physicians have been integrated into the state, and it reflects a series of political struggles and compromises over the powers and prerogatives of physicians, employers, insured persons, and insurance companies.

Regulation of Medicine as a Trade or as a Profession?

Much of the early conflict between doctors and the state in Germany centered on the problem of defining the corporate status of physicians in a society where occupational status needed to be precisely defined. In the United States, where the medical profession and medical technology were both rather highly developed long before there was any widespread acceptance of state intervention in the practice of medicine, the central political issue for physicians has been whether the medical profession would be subject to control by the state at all. In Germany, where the principle of state regulation of occupational associations was already firmly established when medicine first appeared as a fledgling occupation in the late eighteenth and early nineteenth centuries, the central issue was what kind of state control would be applied—regulation of medicine as a trade or as a free profession.

The processes by which occupational groups become accepted as professions within any society are extremely complex. After numerous attempts by scholars to arrive at a precise definition of "profession," most of the current literature agrees on only one point: there can be no precise definition, because recognition of an occupation as a profession is more the result of a political struggle than of some inherent characteristics of the work and the people who perform it. Freidson argues that an occupation gains its special status as a profession because its work is somehow congruent with the beliefs and values of the dominant elite; it is able to persuade the elite that its work is of some special value.[1] The occupation then becomes sponsored by the dominant elite, which uses its political and economic influence to protect the occupation from competition and to foster its development.

Many studies attempt to generalize from the experience of particular professions in order to arrive at a list of necessary steps that a group must follow to become recognized as a profession.[2]

Such lists usually include establishment of schools and definition of a professional body of knowledge; establishment of a code of ethics; establishment of a professional association; and institution of a licensing system controlled by members of the profession. Other studies have shifted their focus from more narrow organizational attributes to the broader social conflicts involved when an occupational group attempts to change its place within the division of labor and the system of social stratification.[3] Magali Larson has analyzed the formation of professions in nineteenth-century Britain and America as a collective effort by broad segments of the new middle class to increase their social mobility through the marketing of new kinds of competence. She demonstrates that both the organizational tactics and the ideological appeals used by new professions were shaped by the broader social conflicts within which professional striving occurred.[4] In Britain and the United States, professions sought to create a market for their services and to produce their services in a way that would be acceptable in a market society.

In Germany, industrialization was accomplished without a complete transformation to a liberal market society,[5] and professions instead were integrated into an older corporatist model of production of services. The struggle of German physicians to achieve the status and privileges of a profession was highly political, with frequent use of labor union strategies, and at times highly legalistic, with use of the courts to establish occupational rights.

For physicians in Germany, the question of whether they were classified as a profession was not purely academic. Since the behavior of all occupational groups and interest associations was regulated by the state, and since regulation differed according to whether the group was thought to be involved in business or in a profession, the decision had important policy consequences. Specifically, the type of regulation applied to physicians (or any other group) would determine the types of taxes paid on earned income, the methods they could use in building and running an interest association, and to some extent, their role in policymaking.

The regulatory instrument for commercial activities was the code of trade. Codes of trade for commercial activities were controls on business practices, such as permissible hours of operation of an enterprise; its number and types of employees; services or products it could sell; limits on the establishment of branch offices and franchises; and requirements for the opening of a new business. In the early nineteenth century, physicians were considered to be small, independent businessmen, and their activities were regulated in the various states by the codes of trade. Gradually, they were granted certain exemptions, notably from the prohibition against strikes and other collective actions, but they sought exemptions from the entire code of trade and regulation through special "physician codes" (*Ärzteordnungen*).[6]

If an occupation were deemed a profession rather than a trade, it would be allowed to regulate itself through a chamber with certain very important privileges. Chambers are organized on a geographical basis, and once an occupation is granted "chamber status," membership in the chamber becomes compulsory for all persons wishing to practice that occupation. In addition, chambers have the right to levy assessments on their members. The right to compel membership as well as financial contributions obviously enables the chambers to build strong interest organizations.

Members of a chamber must abide by its policies. They are specifically forbidden to engage in competition; the very fact that they do not engage in competition is a major rationale for the granting of chamber status. In the case of physicians, chambers regulate the hiring of assistants and replacements, number of office hours, location of officers, formation of group practices, and other conditions of practice. For occupations classified as a profession, the income tax laws grant exemptions from the business profit tax and the turnover tax. Chambers are allowed to establish "honor courts" (*Ehrengerichte*) to regulate misconduct of their members that does not fall under criminal statutes, and the honor courts can issue warnings, censure members, or levy fines. Finally, chambers are required to provide advice to the government on policy issues in their area of competence.[7]

Thus, once an occupational group is granted the status of a profession (or chamber status), it acquires some potent tools for building an interest association (compulsory membership and the right to tax its members) and a legally protected monopoly on the right to promulgate and enforce standards of practice and ethical behavior. Its members acquire substantial protection from competition with each other and with alternative types of practitioners. The chambers are not prohibited from engaging in political activities, despite their role as quasi-governmental agencies and their compulsory membership character, and in fact, are given a special government advisory role on issues that concern them. As will be seen below, physicians' chambers were one major vehicle through which physicians organized and executed their political war with the sickness funds.

Even once the medical profession had been given chamber status in a particular state, the distinction between commercial and professional activities remained an issue. Challenges of one physician by another or by other medical providers were constantly being brought, and issues of the scope of permissible activity were fought out through a series of judicial conflicts. Such conflicts began in the honor courts (if they were intraprofessional disputes), and frequently were decided in the regular court system, or even by the Supreme Court. Typical of these issues was whether physicians were entitled to sell eyeglasses as well as prescribe them. A decision of a Prussian honor court in 1912 stated that the sale of appliances was permissible when it was "harmonious with the practice of medicine," unless the sale involved products which non-doctors sold strictly on a commercial basis, such as eyeglasses.[8] In general, activities which can be performed by businessmen (such as the manufacture and sale of glasses and prosthetic devices) may not be undertaken by physicians. The reasoning behind this principle is that if a doctor does what other people do purely for profit, he would be engaged in business and profitmaking, rather than in the provision of service.[9]

In the mid–nineteenth century, some states and principalities already had specific physician codes that regulated the practice of medicine and conditions of entry into the profession. Physicians' political activities during this period centered on two overriding goals—to assure that physicians would have input into any new legislation or regulations concerning them, and to obtain the right to regulate themselves through occupational chambers. Later, with national unification of the German states and principalities under Prussian leadership, physicians also sought the promulgation of a national law governing physicians to replace the many existing physician codes or codes of trade.

The patterns of physician politics during the nineteenth century seemed to follow those of national politics quite closely. In the 1840s, a period of Liberalism characterized by formation of new interest groups with demands for parliamentary democracy, national unification, and more popular participation in policymaking, physicians were engaging in parallel activities. Numerous local and regional medical congresses were held, and many medical associations were formed. They generally called for formation of a unified professional organization based on democratic self-governing principles and for greater participation of physician associations in the formation of laws and regulations affecting medical practice.[10]

The platform of the Congress of Saxon Physicians in 1848 is illustrative of some of these concerns. The demands included formation of physicians' committees with honor courts and arbitration commissions; formation of a physicians' chamber, elected entirely by physician members, to work with state health agencies in drafting medical legislation; establishment of hospitals and standardized medical facilities throughout the country; standardized provisions for medical licensure, including a more flexible medical curriculum and state licensing examinations to be taken after one year of hospital internship; and replacement of the system of separate classes of doctors distinguished by their academic degrees with a unified, single class of physicians.[11]

Similar demands were made by a conference of Prussian physicians convened by the Prussian regime in 1848 to aid it in reforming medical legislation. The conference called for a unified medical profession, limitation of the practice of healing arts to licensed physicians, requirement of a Gymnasium certificate and university degree for a medical license, freedom to establish medical practices in a place of the physician's choice, and formation of professional honor courts.[12] In general, the physicians were concerned with establishing a national organization and standardizing the various laws governing physicians in the German states and principalities. They wanted to standardize education and licensing requirements and keep unlicensed healers from practicing medicine. These demands for more physician control over entry into the profession and standards of practice were to continue as a major object of physician politics for several decades.

The general Conservative reaction in Germany during the 1850s was reflected in the waning of political activity among physicians' associations. The associations practically stopped meeting, many went out of existence, and the frequent convening of congresses and conferences of the past decade came to a halt. Many states which had earlier allowed or solicited physician participation in policymaking returned to strict regulation of physicians promulgated from above. Prussia introduced a provision into its criminal code that obligated physicians to provide medical services (the so-called Paragraph 200). Some states even went so far as to make private physicians directly responsible to a state health agency or to the city police department. Then, during the 1860s, there was some liberalization in policies toward physicians, with several states allowing physicians to form chambers with honor courts, or to elect physician representatives to the state legislative bodies.[13]

The most important change of the preunification period was the amendment of the Prussian Code of Trade as applied to physicians. The main issues were the right to settle and open a practice without special permits, the obligation of physicians to provide medical care (Paragraph 200), and the status of unlicensed physicians. The last issue, euphemistically called "therapeutic freedom" (*Kurierfreiheit*), was at bottom a question of whether the government would support physicians' demands to outlaw the provision of health care by assorted groups of natural and other healers. The Prussian parliament in 1869 granted physicians the right to settle wherever they wished, and eliminated the hated Paragraph 200, but refused to accept an amendment that would prevent unlicensed physicians from practicing. When national unification occurred in 1871, the Prussian Code of Trade then became the code for the entire nation.[14]

The unification of the German states under Bismarck's leadership gave new impetus for a national physicians' organization. Two years later, in 1873, the Deutsche Ärtzevereinsbund (DÄV) was formed as a national union of medical associations. Its leader was Hermann Eberhard Richter, a physician who had been "on the barricades" in 1848. Membership in the association was open only to medical societies and not to individual doctors. The stated purposes of the DÄV were to further the art and science of medicine, to engage in public health care, and to influence health legislation. In order to belong, a medical association was required to share these goals and to be actively striving for official state recognition of a physician organization in its region.[15] Membership in the organization grew rapidly; upon its formation in 1873, 84 of the existing 170 medical associations joined. By 1894, the DÄV claimed 239 member associations, representing sixty-two percent of all physicians; by 1927 that figure was ninty-five percent.[16]

The DÄV was governed by an annual general assembly of delegates from the member medical associations, and a small executive committee. The leadership perceived the role of the association as promoting professional interests (*Standesinteresse*), rather than purely economic ones. Thus, the overriding goal of the DÄV was to promote a national physicians' code and to secure chamber status for the profession nationwide. Despite constant pressure by the DÄV, the national government refused to create a national physicians' code, and insisted instead that regulation of medical practice was the responsibility of the different states. Eventually, several of the states did grant chamber status to their physicians—Prussia in 1887, Oldenburg in 1891, Bavaria in 1895, Anhalt in 1900, Lübeck in 1903, Lippe Detmold in 1921, Württemberg in 1925, and Thuringia in 1926.[17]

It was not until 1935 that a national physicians' code was finally achieved. This first code, from which the current Federal Physicians' Code (*Bundesärzteordnung*) is derived, declared that medicine is not a trade, but by its very nature a free profession.[18] The question of professional status of physicians was thus not completely resolved until the 1930s, when, incidentally, the other major issues of physicians-government relationships were also resolved by a series of government orders.

It should be stressed that the organization of the medical profession into chambers does not distinguish it from many other professions, such as lawyers, tax advisers, pharmacists, and architects, for which there are chambers with similar authority. In all cases, the chambers set out codes of behavior and rules of competition and enforce them with full governmental authority. Physicians' benefits from and obligations to the state may differ from those of other occupations in substance, but they are embodied in political institutions whose form and functions are similar. The issue of the special status of the medical profession was thus settled in a way that distinguished it from other occupations only slightly. The medical profession had its own chambers and certain rules which applied uniquely to the practice of medicine. But the basic character of the state's regulation of the profession through self-governing chambers whose decisions were ultimately subordinate to the national legislative and judicial organs rendered the medical profession politically analogous to numerous other occupational groups.

The Rights of Physicians as Employees

Beyond the fundamental problem of defining the corporate status of the medical profession, another important issue for physicians was the definition of employment relations between physicians and sickness funds, and between physicians and state agencies, such as public health agencies, municipal hospitals, and prisons.

Over this issue of employment conditions, physicians in Germany formed trade unions and through collective action were able to force both sickness funds and government to make important concessions.

In order to understand the issue of job security, one must understand the structure of medical practice during the nineteenth century. There were essentially three kinds of practice for physicians:

1. *An entirely private office practice for patients without membership in a sickness fund.* The number of these practices was sometimes limited (by the regional chambers), so that a doctor could not open an office merely at his own will. Young doctors for the most part obtained a practice by purchasing one of a retired or deceased doctor. Even where the establishment of new practices was not limited by law, it was often very difficult for a new physician to break in.

2. *Office practice for members of sickness funds.* In order to establish such a practice, the physician had to be hired by the individual sickness fund on the basis of a private contract. Some funds (the Miners' Fund and Railroad Workers' Fund) hired a single physician for all of their members in a given district. Most funds used a closed panel system, offering their members a limited choice of physicians with whom the fund had contracted.[19] But in either case, the funds deliberately limited the number of physicians they hired, because the fund administrators believed that limiting the availability of physicians to members was important to keep costs down. The result for physicians was that sickness fund jobs were difficult to obtain.

3. *Employment by municipal hospitals, charity hospitals, public health agencies, prisons, military organizations, shipping companies, or mining companies.* Under such an arrangement, the physician was hired as a salaried employee. It is important to note that there was no sector of private, for-profit hospitals in Germany; almost all hospitals were run by municipalities as public agencies.

Although the number of salaried employment positions (with sickness funds, hospitals, and other agencies) was limited and only a minority of physicians were so employed, the issue of employment conditions and job security gained importance for two main reasons. First, health insurance through sickness funds was steadily expanding, so that the trend was for more and more physicians to be employed by them. Second, the number of physicians was growing rapidly (from about 15,000 in 1880 to about 27,000 in 1900),[20] so that there was increased competition for the few secure jobs that did exist. Sickness funds had the upper hand, both because they operated in a sellers' market (there were more physicians willing to take fund jobs than jobs available), and because they contracted individually with each physician.

For employed physicians, the chief areas of conflict centered on the terms of their contracts with their employers, including length of time needed for notice of termination of contract by the employer; length of time needed for notice of termination of contract by the physician; grounds for dismissal; provisions for arbitration of disputes; level of payment; mode of payment. Employed physicians felt that they held their jobs at the whim of the sickness fund directors. Professional newspapers were full of stories of physicians being dismissed by the funds for capricious or arbitrary reasons—for temporary inability to work due to an accident, for personal disagreements or conflicts with a director, for political views—or simply dismissed with no grounds given at all.[21] The conflict between physicians and their employers over job security was exacerbated by the physicians' perception of fund directors' lower social status:

> It must be emphasized that the fund directors are Social Democrats and blue-collar workers, and thereby the social inferiors of doctors; thus such people occupy a position as leaders and employers of doctors, whereas they would otherwise in life be considered dependent on the bourgeoisie. Certainly many doctors see them [the fund directors] as subordinates as a matter of right.[22]

Initially, the political struggles of physicians against their employers were carried out through the chambers, where chambers existed. In order to protect themselves, physicians created commissions to oversee employment contracts (*Vertragskommissionen*).[23] The formal authority of these commissions varied in the individual states. In some, the power to regulate contracts was expressly granted to the chambers; in some, the right to regulate contracts was implicitly granted; in other states, the power to regulate contracts was provisionally granted to independent interest associations of physicians; and in still others, the independent physicians' associations assumed the function of regulating contracts without any state authority.

The contract commissions had no formal authority to coerce physicians, but by tying their activities to the codes of ethics and coordinating their activities with local medical associations, they were often able to gain concessions from the employers. The commissions reviewed contracts between physicians and employers and would approve only those that were in accordance with their own "principles." By 1913 most contracts contained a provision that they would become effective only on approval of the relevant commission. The principles included the proper procedure for termination of a contract; minimum notice periods for both sides; provisions for arbitration of disputes by formal courts of arbitration; prohibition against a doctor's accepting an honorarium of less than the standard prevailing rate or than he had previously earned; prohibition against his accepting a salary in a position where reimbursement had previously been by fee-for-service; and prohibition against accepting a position at a hospital or other facility where unlicensed practitioners were employed. Physicians were asked to sign a declaration of acceptance of the principles of the contract commission (a so-called *Revers*). If a physician signed such a declaration, he was considered to have given his word "on his honor." Breach of honor was grounds for an ethical charge and summons before the honor court, which would eventually publish its findings and the names of any offenders.

What means did the commissions have to induce the physicians to sign such declarations or abide by their principles? First, the chambers' codes of ethics often included a requirement that the physician have commission approval before making any oral or written contract with a sickness fund, hospital, clinic, or other public or private institution. Thus, even though commissions were only committees of the chambers, chambers could enforce cooperation with them by making cooperation part of their codes of ethics. Since membership in the chambers was compulsory, physicians were ultimately forced to accept the policies of the contract commissions. Second, the local medical societies often made the declaration of acceptance of principles a condition for membership. Other societies did not make the declaration compulsory, but strongly recommended that physicians sign it. And finally some chambers made the declaration a condition for voting privileges in the chamber.

The contract commissions used their power against state government authorities as well as sickness funds. They engaged in battles over physicians' contracts with the postal service sickness fund, railroad administration, and prisons. When a state authority refused to accept the contract principles of a commission, the commission tried to boycott the agency by discouraging all doctors from contracting with it. Although state govermnents had the formal authority to regulate the activities of the commissions (through their authority to regulate the chambers), they rarely interfered, even when the commissions were opposing other government agencies. The government's reluctance to interfere was due to its perception that the doctors could and would form contract commissions outside the chambers (i.e., within the independent medical associations). Were this to happen (as it had in several areas), the government would have no formal authority over the commissions. Where the commissions were committees of the chambers, the government at least had the right to supervise activities of the chamber as a whole, however weak that right might be in practice.

Although the contract commissions were active in protecting physicians against the sickness funds and state agencies, there was no unified political organization of physicians until 1900. In that year, the Leipziger Verband was formed as a trade union organization for physicians; its full title was the "Union of German Physicians for the Defense of Their Economic Interests" (Verband der Ärtze Deutschlands zur Wahrung ihrer wirtschaftlichen Interessen). It was generally called the Leipziger Verband (LV) after the city where it originated, or the Hartmannbund (HB) after its principal founder and leader.

Several factors precipitated the formation of the LV. First, many physicians perceived a decline in their economic status, especially since the introduction of compulsory health insurance. Not only did they resent their dependence on the sickness funds, but they also felt that the sickness funds were depressing their earnings. Relative to those of other professions with similar social status (e.g., an *Oberlehrer* or Gymnasium teacher), physicians' incomes seemed to have declined.

Second, many physicians were losing faith in the ability of the DÄV to protect their economic interests. The DÄV restricted its activities largely to drafting and circulation of memoranda and petitions on the questions of a national physicians' code and chamber status, and was not willing to engage in more aggressive tactics. It eschewed electoral politics, maintained a position of formal neutrality toward the different parties, and refused to use its funds to help enable physicians to leave their practices while they served in the state or national parliaments.[24]

The internal organization of the DÄV was hardly suited to protecting the economic interests of the profession. Since the executive committee was composed of members scattered throughout the Empire and authoritative policy could be made only by the annual (or at most semiannual) assembly, aggressive, quick decisionmaking and responsiveness to numerous problems arising in the various states were impossible. Moreover, because the majority of physicians were not employed by funds or other organizations, the delegates to the DÄV assembly were more concerned with opening up sickness fund practice to all physicians than with protecting the jobs and working conditions of the currently employed physicians.[25] Leaders of the new Leipziger Verband, including its founder, openly accused the DÄV of neglecting the economic interests of physicians and of allowing the sickness funds to obtain a monopoly position.

A third factor was the challenge to the medical profession posed by the Socialists. The Social Democratic Party and its newspaper, *Vorwärts*, generally sided with the sickness funds in conflicts between physicians and funds, because the funds were perceived as organs of worker participation and as organizations that benefited working people directly. In 1901, part of the official platform of the Social Democratic Party was a demand for free medical services, and Socialist groups at various times called for nationalization or socialization of physicians.[26]

One Socialist physician, Dr. Landmann, developed a system of medical practice based on Socialist ideas and was able to persuade many sickness funds to adopt it.[27] Landmann believed that physicians maintained their high economic and social position by tricking the proletariat into thinking illness was caused by normal environmental factors rather than by the economic structure of society. His basic idea was to make medical care more efficient by organizing clinics along the lines of large industry. Each physician was to be obligated to make his instruments available for use by the clinic; although the physician owned his instruments, the fund was to be responsible for repairs and therefore would own any replacement parts it provided. Physicians would be required to be on call and available for emergency care outside the regular clinic hours, and to be on duty during Sundays and afternoons on a rotating schedule. They would be pressured to reduce the number of prescriptions and hospital referrals; in Landmann's model contract, the number of referrals was limited to the average of the previous three years and if exceeded, the physicians would have to pay twenty percent of the extra cost out of their own salaries. Physicians were to receive their housing from each sickness fund, and to be forbidden to change their housing arrangements without the permission of the fund directors.

In 1898 Dr. Landmann tried to introduce his system in the town of Barmen. He began by trying to bring the local pharmacists under the control of the sickness funds, so that drugs would be produced in pharmacies owned by the funds. The funds asked the physicians to declare their solidarity with this endeavor, and when the physicians refused they were fired and replaced by doctors brought in from outside. The conflict resulted in a doctors' strike that lasted eight days, whereupon the government intervened and concluded a more favorable contract with the physicians. A few similar strikes occurred in other towns where the Landmann system was introduced. These strikes all generated wide publicity in both the national press and the medical press, and even *Vorwärts* editorialized in favor of the physicians, who, the paper said, now resembled workers.[28] Discussions of these events in the medical press led to a famous exchange in which a Dr. Warmiensis (a pen name) called for all physicians simultaneously to terminate their contracts with sickness funds and to treat all patients henceforth as private patients. Dr. Hartmann, in an open reply to Dr. Warmiensis, called on physicians to organize themselves and to build a "strike fund" by collecting one mark from every physician each week.[29]

Hartmann founded the Leipziger Verband a few months later with only twenty-one physicians. Its membership remained extremely small at first. In the first three years it had around two thousand members, out of about thirty thousand physicians, while the DÄV represented about three hundred associations with over eighteen thousand individual members at about the same time.[30] After 1903, membership grew dramatically (see table 3.1). Plaut credits the growth to a series of very successful strikes staged by the LV in 1903, and the attendant publicity. But it is clear that the union leaders also adopted some very strategic policies to build up the membership. Hartmann decided to tone down the union rhetoric used in his speeches and publications, in order not to keep away physicians who felt it improper for physicians to join a labor organization. The LV leaders realized they needed the cooperation of the DÄV, and in 1903 the LV agreed to become formally an "economic department" of the DÄV. Although they still remained essentially separate organizations, the DÄV now encouraged its members to join the LV as individuals. LV organizers went into hospitals and medical schools to recruit students and junior physicians, and lowered the dues for these groups to half price.[31]

Most important for organization building, the LV leadership provided a variety of selective incentives for physicians to join. The leaders used members' dues and even took out loans to create a credit union, a widows' fund, a pension fund, and a burial fund.[32] The union also set up a placement service for physicians

Table 3.1 Members of the Leipziger Verband as a Percentage of
All Physicians

Year	Percent
1903 (July)	6%
1903 (August)	31
1904	53
1905	56
1906	61
1907	63
1908	70
1909	70
1910	71
1911	72
1913	75
1919	90
1925	88
1927	84

Sources: 1903–11: Theodor Plaut, *Der Gewerkschaftskampf der Deutschen Ärtze* (Karlsrühe: G. Braunsche, 1913), p. 97, based on annual business reports of the Leipziger Verband.
1913–27: Heinz Schmitt, *Entstehung und Wandlungen der Zielsetzungen, der Struktur und der Wirkungen der Berufsverbände* (Berlin: Duncker and Humblot, 1966), p. 59.

(*Stellenvermittlung*), through which it arranged sales of private practices and maintained lists of open positions in hospitals, funds, public agencies, and shipping companies. A total of around two thousand jobs a year were handled by the union between 1904 and 1911.[33] The placement service directly benefited physicians because it was less costly and more honest than the alternative commercial services, which charged thirty to fifty percent of the yearly income of the practice as a sales commission, and therefore had an incentive to misrepresent its financial position. The union provided the service at cost and had an incentive to be honest. If it misled a doctor into buying a practice in an area where competition was already strong, it would lose not only his allegiance but also that of the local doctors who would resent the added competition.

The Leipziger Verband enjoyed enormous success in its first years. Between 1900 and 1911, it engaged in about two hundred conflicts per year and won about ninety percent of them.[34] The main tactics of the LV were the strike and the boycott. When an employer refused to grant conditions demanded by the physicians, or treated a physician unfairly, the LV organized a collective strike. If necessary, a boycott was also organized to prevent the employer from bringing in strikebreaking physicians from outside, and the names of blacklisted employers were publicized through the medical newspapers. The annual report of the LV for 1909–10 reports that 947 boycotts were organized in that year alone.[35]

The union had several instruments for maintaining solidarity with its strikes and boycotts. It used part of its substantial funds to create strike funds to support physicians while they were on strike, and to advertise boycotts of the blacklisted employers. The placement service was also useful for maintaining physician solidarity during strikes; physicians who might otherwise be willing to act as strikebreakers could be offered jobs in other areas. The LV organized "offensive and defensive alliances" (*Schutz- und Trutzbündnisse*) during strikes, which were pacts among the physicians not to sign an individual contract with an employer who was being struck.

Through the contract commissions, the chambers, and the Leipziger Verband, physicians were basically successful in achieving better job security, working conditions, and higher fees, and in resisting the efforts of the sickness funds and municipal agencies to socialize the medical profession. While much of their success should be attributed to their strong organizing ability, their strong bargaining position derived from the method by which the government chose to guarantee health services. The national program required that sickness funds provide service benefits, not cash or indemnity benefits, so that the funds were virtually required to contract with physicians.

The tremendous success rate of physician strikes only confirms the structural weakness of the funds in the system. The strong collective organization of physicians eventually prompted the formation of interest associations of sickness funds—in 1894, the General Union of Sickness Funds (representing local funds); in 1907, the Union of Factory Funds; in 1910, the General Union of Guild Funds; in 1912, the General Union of German Sickness Funds; and in 1914, the Imperial Union of German Agricultural Funds.[36] But the high number of strikes and boycotts was also indicative of the instability of the system. As the government's compulsory health insurance program grew, the question of the right of sickness funds to limit their physician panels became more acute for both funds and doctors, as did the right of sickness funds to control the practice of their physicians. A dispute resolution mechanism more stable than the strike-and-settle model of the early 1900s was still missing.

Stabilizing the Relationship between Sickness Funds and Physicians

Because of government mandated health insurance, physicians and government came into conflict over the scope and organization of the public sector of medicine, that is, the services provided to publicly insured patients through sickness funds. Physicians battled most directly with the sickness funds, because the funds, as bodies of public law, were given wide latitude in setting their own policies. But eventually the government was forced to referee the conflict, because an impasse between the funds and the physicians was politically intolerable.

The government's national health insurance program was undoubtedly the most important factor that shaped the relationship between physicians and sickness funds. Although sickness funds had existed before the introduction of national health insurance, the social insurance legislation of 1883 gave a big impetus to the growth of sickness funds and ultimately increased physicians' dependence on funds as sources of employment. The program began small, but grew steadily. Only eleven percent of the population were covered in 1888, but by 1900 seventeen percent were covered, and by 1910 about twenty percent.[37] This steady growth in the proportion of population included in the public program was accomplished through two legislative mechanisms. First, Parliament passed a series of increases in the minimum income level necessary for exemption from the compulsory program. Second, it gradually extended insurance to more social categories of people.

Because the original public health insurance program was so small, existing medical associations greeted it with verbal hostility but little organized protest. Prominent physicians argued that doctors were the natural allies of the poor and that the lower classes were best served by a "free profession" with a free choice of doctors. The house organ of the only national professional association, the Deutsche Ärztevereinsbund, clung to an image of the private system of medicine as one in which "every suffering person could find medical help at a price corresponding to his financial means."[38] Apparently the Health Insurance Act of 1883 was passed with no input from professional organizations, and the new program was not even discussed in professional journals until after it had already passed.[39]

The medical profession found itself in a contradictory position vis-à-vis the insurance system. On the one hand, physicians felt their professional and economic freedom was jeopardized by the intrusion of government into the doctor-patient relationship. In particular, private physicians (i.e., ones not admitted to fund practice) saw the expansion of insurance as a reduction of their market. The more patients that were included in the public sector by virtue of compulsory insurance, the fewer patients there would be in the private sector. Undoubtedly physicians felt the contraction of the private market all the more keenly because the number of physicians was expanding rapidly during the same period. Although there are no definitive manpower statistics, it seems clear from the estimates of medical historians that the ratio of population to physicians declined dramatically in the twenty years following the introduction and expansion of compulsory insurance—from three thousand people per doctor in 1883, to two thousand per doctor in 1913.[40]

The professional journals did not discuss the tighter market, however. Instead, they stressed "free choice of doctor" as the important issue. Since each sickness fund would reimburse only physicians with whom it had contracts, fund patients were restricted to that group of doctors. The professional associations argued that this restriction of public patients' choice of physician was an infringement of personal rights as well as a hindrance to a good doctor-patient relationship.

In effect, social insurance created two patient pools where there had formerly been one. The creation of two separate markets for health services had a strong influence on the development of medical politics. Physicians were in the ironic position of trying to restrict the size of the public sector (and thus preserve the private sector) and to increase their access to it at the same time. Since neither the DÄV nor the LV engaged very much in electoral politics, and physicians had few representatives in Parliament, the medical profession was not in a position to fight legislative initiatives for expansion of health insurance. (One exception to this pattern was a physician strike staged in Remscheid to protest the elevation of the minimum income level from 10,000 to 15,000 marks in 1920.)[41] Professional associations therefore turned their attention to expanding physicians' access to the pool of insured patients.

But even on the question of increasing physician access to publicly insured patients, insurance doctors and private doctors had divergent interests. Thus, at various times and in various places, physicians' organizations were apt to take either side of the issue on the question of "free choice of doctor." One study of physicians' associations in 1904 found that in 24 of 173 associations, official policy was against free choice of doctor, because the physicians themselves were "satisfied" with their relationships with the funds.[42] But overall, as the government expanded the compulsory health insurance program, more and more physicians supported the free choice principle. Ultimately, the primary goal of the Leipziger Verband came to be achieving the right of all doctors to be admitted to insurance practice.

In 1911, the government issued a proposal to expand the public health insurance program yet another time, amend existing program regulations, and codify them into the Imperial Insurance Code (RVO). The proposed RVO, to take effect on January 1, 1914, would be harmful to physician interests in two significant ways. It would expand the population covered to nearly thirty percent. And, for the first time, the law would allow sickness funds to give cash (or indemnity) benefits instead of medical services.[43] This provision would clearly reduce some of the pressure on the funds to settle with physicians during strikes. These changes were counterbalanced by a provision that healers without academic training and formal licensure could no longer treat fund patients. But physicians saw a threat to their position in the proposal, and in October 1913, in an extraordinary session, the general assembly of the DÄV called for a general strike.

At this point, the government stepped in to mediate between the funds and the physicians, and the result was the historic Berlin Treaty of 1913. The parties to the treaty were the DÄV and Leipziger Verband, representing physicians, and the Union for Defense of the Interests of Factory Sickness Funds, General Union of German Sickness Funds, and the Union of German Local Sickness Funds on the other side.[44] The Berlin Treaty was the first victory for physicians in their fight to gain access to the public sector, but it was by no means complete. Instead of requiring sickness funds to admit all doctors to insurance practice, the agreement required the funds to maintain a certain ratio of doctors to fund members (initially, 1:1,350).

The real importance of the Berlin Treaty is that it was an initial attempt to establish regular procedures for negotiating the conflicting interests of physicians and sickness fund administrators. The treaty established various committees on which physicians and funds had equal representation. An admissions committee had authority to set the physician/insured person ratio and to select future physicians for admission to insurance practice. A contract committee was responsible for setting basic guidelines for the contracts between individual physicians and sickness funds. Finally, an arbitration committee composed of representatives of the government's insurance commission, the sickness funds, and physicians was established to handle conflicts that could not be resolved in the other committees.[45]

Relations between the funds and the physicians were generally peaceful for the next several years, particularly during World War I. The Berlin Treaty was to be effective for ten years, but tensions over the level of physicians' fees, for which the treaty had no provisions, led to its dissolution. Again physicians began to conduct strikes, and both sides terminated the agreement. From this point on, the role of the government changed from mediator to regulator. During the next decade, the government issued a series of emergency orders in 1923, 1930, and 1931 that dramatically changed the character of sickness fund–physician relationships and shaped the countervailing power model on which today's system is based.

The essence of the emergency orders was to consolidate physicians into large bargaining units, and also to strengthen the ability of sickness funds to control utilization of services. Consolidation of physicians' power occurred through two means. First, the regulations mandated formation of regional associations of insurance doctors (AIDs), with the status of bodies of public law. Physicians who were admitted to insurance practice were required to join their regional AID. Second, the new regulations eliminated individual contracts between sickness funds and physicians and substituted a system of collective contracts between the funds and the AIDs.[46] These collective contracts would then be "recognized" by each individual physician wishing to be admitted to insurance practice. The regulations also increased physician access to the pool of publicly insured patients by raising to 1:600 the physician/insured person ratio.[47]

As bodies of public law, the AIDs were charged with assuring the medical care of the insurance fund members and their dependents. This provision, sometimes called the *Sicherstellungsauftrag* (see RVO sec. 368n, pt. 1), has turned out to be a potent weapon for the office-based insurance doctors. They have used it to maintain a virtual monopoly on the provision of ambulatory health services to insured persons.

The regulations which created the associations of insurance doctors stipulated that these organizations should be able to represent the economic interests of physicians in the strongest possible manner. Because the Hartmannbund (as the LV was now called) was the stongest professional association with a regional organizational structure, it was able to control the executive committees of the new AIDs.[48] This meant that the professional association which had originally been formed to resist outside control of health services, and specifically of physician employment, was now actually invested with public authority; the Hartmannbund, through its control of the insurance doctors' associations, had in effect become a part of the government administration of health services. The Hartmannbund still exists as a separate, voluntary interest association, but its ties to the AIDs are extremely close.

The series of emergency orders also strengthened the hand of sickness funds considerably. First, the orders established a method of paying physicians which made them bear some of the financial risks of the insurance system. Under this method, each sickness fund paid the AID a fixed pool of money, established on a capitation basis, which the AID then distributed to its members. This method was eventually modified substantially, but the outlines of the system were preserved, so that some degree of fixed budgeting could still be reestablished in the 1970s (see chapters 5 and 6). Second, sickness funds were given authority to monitor and control physicians' therapeutic decisions. The funds were allowed to set standards of "necessary and economical" treatment, to monitor actual procedures and prescriptions, and to hold physicians liable for the costs of those deemed excessive. Funds were also allowed to require a second opinion on any decisions to grant patients wage continuation payments. (These controls are examined in chapters 7 and 8.)

One can never completely account for the power of a social group. But it seems clear from this history that the idea that the medical profession's political strength derives entirely from its special status as a profession or from its monopoly on technical expertise must be dismissed. Since self-regulation within a broad, legislatively mandated framework is the norm for occupational groups in Germany, the pattern of professional self-regulation by physicians cannot be interpreted as any kind of special privilege granted by the state. Nevertheless, the general pattern of allowing interests to form chambers—with all the powers that implies—certainly benefited physicians in forming a political organization and maintaining a monoply on health services.

The trade union activities of the medical profession, however, were clearly of major significance in the development of the political strength of physicians relative to other important organizations with whom they deal. The government's sponsorship of public health insurance through sickness funds offering service benefits increased physicians' dependence on employment by the funds, but also gave added strenghth to the physician trade union movement. Had the government chosen to socialize health services (and thus become a monopoly employer) or to provide cash benefits which patients could use to purchase services in a private market, physicians' organizations would have had less bargaining power.

What seems to have happened is that certain explicit government decisions created a system of concentrated physician organizations with legal authority to negotiate exclusively with sickness funds and to administer certain parts of the health insurance program. In a sense, the government's solution to the problem of controlling a group with a monopoly on valued technical expertise was to make the group more powerful, but to confront it with an equally powerful opponent. Regardless of whether the strategy was successful, the history of the development of the current system demonstrates that societal decisions about organizing group relationships are of crucial significance in the creation of collective power.

Physicians have a kind of power that is not adequately captured by an analysis of the collective actions of the medical profession. They make a variety of discretionary decisions that, in the aggregate, strongly influence the implementation of a public health insurance program. They decide on the services to provide and recommend in their own offices, and they allocate referrals to specialists and hospital physicians. They also prescribe and authorize government reimbursement for drugs, appliances, and various supplementary therapies. In the West German national health insurance system, physicians also preside over an enormous cash transfer program for temporarily disabled workers. These decisions are directly *allocative* decisions.

The mix and volume of services that are provided by the health care system are in turn influenced by another range of discretionary decisions by individual physicians—about whether and how to specialize, which sector to enter (office-based, hospital-based, public health service, occupational medicine, and so on), where to locate one's practice, how to equip and staff one's office, and how much time to put into various aspects of one's job. In the West German system, with its guild traditions, these "second order" decisions have been more heavily regulated than in the United States. Before proceeding with a discussion of allocative authority of physicians, it will be useful to have some idea of the number and kinds of physicians that constitute the West German medical profession, and the factors that influence the structure of the profession.

The Structure of the Medical Profession

West Germany has one of the highest physician-to-population ratios in the world. In 1976, there were about 122,000 active physicians for a population of about 61 million, giving a ratio of about 198 physicians for every 100,000 people. In Western Europe, only Austria has a higher ratio. In the United States in 1976, there were about 350,000 active physicians and about 173 physicians for every 100,000 people.

As is true for the United States, national figures on the supply of physicians disguise severe discrepancies across different geographic areas. Physician density of the different states in 1976 varied from 167 physicians per 100,000 people in Lower Saxony to 342 per 100,000 in West Berlin.[1] And, of course, the differences are even more severe between smaller areas. The density of office-based physicians in the 58 planning regions varies from about 62 per 100,000 to 135 per 100,000.[2]

To enter the medical profession in West Germany, a physician must be licensed, as in the United States. Licenses are technically granted by the appropriate health or social affairs ministry of each *Land*, but in practice medical licensure is controlled by the physician chamber of each *Land*.[3] In this context, the chambers have been called "the long arm of the *Land* ministry."[4] A license to practice, though granted by an individual *Land*, is valid for the entire country. In the United States, by contrast, licenses are valid only in the state in which they are issued; most states have reciprocal agreements for recognition of licenses, however.

Sectors of Practice. Compared with the American medical profession, the West German medical profession is segmented into rather rigid occupational groups, each with legally defined rights to practice certain kinds of medicine. Again, this structural characteristic of the profession stems from the corporatist tradition of rigidly dividing work roles among guilds. The most important division is between office-based and hospital-based physicians. (This particular division characterizes most European medical systems and is not unique to Germany.) Other major subgroups within the profession are public health service physicians (employed by state and local agencies), occupational physicians (employed by factories and large businesses), and control doctors (employed by sickness funds). Physicians in these branches of employment are not allowed to have private practices, or to provide general care to the patients they treat in the course of their duties. (For example, an occupational physician may treat injuries that occur on the job, but may not also provide primary care to the employees of his employer.)

Hospital-based physicians are salaried employees of a hospital and cannot practice medicine outside it, even to provide follow-up care for patients they have treated in the hospital or to perform preadmission diagnostic workups. Office-based physicians, unlike their American counterparts, rarely have staff privileges in local hospitals, and may provide only ambulatory care. There are a few exceptions to these rules. Hospital chiefs of staff, who comprise about six percent of hospital physicians, are allowed to maintain a private fee-for-service practice on the side as well as provide ambulatory care for members of sickness funds. A small number of office-based physicians, particularly in some

Table 4.1 Staff Privileges of West German Physicians

	1960	1974	1975	1976
Belegsärzte (MDs with staff privileges)	7,368	4,502	4,878	5,166
Total office-based physicians	46,654	50,731	50,098	51,045
Proportion of MDs with staff privileges	15.8%	8.0%	9.7%	10.1%

Sources: 1960–74: Calculated from Theo Siebeck, *Zur Kostenentwicklung in der Krankenversicherung* (Bonn: Bundesverband der Ortskrankenkassen, 1976), p. 73; and Statistiches Bundesamt, *Statistiches Jahrbuch für die Bundesrepublik Deutschland*, annual volumes. 1975–76: Calculated from Klaus Gehb, "Die ärztliche Versorgung in der Bundesrepublik Deutschland," *Deutsches Ärzteblatt* 19 (1976), table 3. These figures do *not* include West Berlin.

specialties (ophthalmology, ear, nose, and throat, and obstetrics-gynecology), are allowed to see their patients in both their office and a hospital. As can be seen in table 4.1, the number of physicians with staff privileges is small both absolutely and proportionately, and until very recently there has been a definite trend away from staff privileges and the consequent integration of the ambulatory and hospital sectors.

The most striking trend in the recent development of the West German medical profession is the shift from fee-for-service office-based practice to salaried hospital-based practice (see table 4.2). The absolute number of office-based physicians has grown only slightly over the past two decades, and the ratio of office-based physicians to population has remained relatively constant. In contrast, the absolute number of hospital-based physicians has nearly tripled and the ratio of hospital-based physicians to population has more than doubled.

Table 4.3 presents a comparison of the sector sizes in West Germany and the United States. The figures must be treated with some caution, however. Because of the strict legal separation of the two sectors in Germany, the classification of physicians as "office-based" and "hospital-based" does not have the same meaning there as in the United States. In the German data, any physician in the ambulatory sector (*niedergelassene Arzt*) is automatically office-based regardless of whether he also has staff privileges at a hospital. Likewise, the hospital chiefs of staff, who are allowed to provide outpatient care in a private practice, do not count as office-based, though they might spend more time delivering outpatient than inpatient care. In the United States data,

Table 4.2 Active Physicians in West Germany

Year	Total Number Per 100,000 Inhab- itants	Office-Based Total Number	Office-Based Number Per 100,000 Inhab- itants	Hospital-Based Total Number	Hospital-Based Number Per 100,000 Inhab- itants	Administrative* Total Number	Administrative* Number Per 10,000 Inhab- itants
1955	136.5	42,382	85.6	20,136	40.7	5,084	10.3
1956	135.6	43,466	85.0	20,411	39.9	5,440	10.6
1957	136.2	44,072	85.0	20,709	40.0	5,884	11.3
1958	135.3	44,733	85.2	20,395	38.9	5,908	11.3
1959	137.2	45,124	85.1	21,023	39.6	6,638	12.5
1960	138.8	46,654	86.8	21,142	39.3	6,807	12.7
1961	142.2	49,790	88.0	22,966	40.6	8,069	14.3
1962	143.4	50,476	88.2	23,336	40.8	8,285	14.5
1963	143.5	50,375	87.1	24,136	41.7	8,514	14.7
1964	143.7	50,060	85.4	25,324	43.2	8,819	15.1
1965	144.7	50,215	84.7	26,535	44.7	9,051	15.3
1966	145.0	49,945	83.5	27,622	46.2	9,133	15.3
1967	147.7	49,940	83.3	28,985	48.3	9,634	16.1
1968	150.3	50,178	83.0	30,916	51.1	9,788	16.2
1969	153.5	50,379	82.3	33,770	55.2	9,785	16.0
1970	163.4	50,731	83.2	38,655	63.4	10,268	16.8
1971	169.0	51,159	83.2	42,245	68.7	10,506	17.1
1972	173.8	51,778	83.8	45,138	73.0	10,487	17.0
1973	179.0	52,473	84.6	47,698	77.0	10,809	17.4
1974	185.0	53,873	86.8	50,341	81.1	10,447	16.8
1975	193.0	55,692	90.0	52,371	84.7	10,663	17.2
1976	198.3	56,969	92.6	54,513	88.6	10,593	17.2
1977	204.2	58,222	94.8	56,334	91.7	10,718	17.5
1978	212.0	59,036	96.2	59,183	96.5	11,814	19.3

Note: *Administrative physicians are those employed in public health agencies, bodies of public law, research institutes, and private enterprise (including factory doctors).
Source: Statistisches Bundesamt, *Statistisches Jahrbuch für die Bundesrepublik Deutschland*, annual volumes.

Table 4.3 Distribution of Active Physicians by Activity: United States and West Germany, 1976

Activity	Percent of Active Physicians West Germany	Percent of Active Physicians U.S.
Office-based	46.7%	62.1%
Hospital-based	44.7	29.2
Administration or research	8.7	8.6

Sources: Statistisches Bundesamt, *Statistisches Jahrbuch für die Bundesrepublik Deutschland 1978*, table 17.10; American Medical Association, *Profile of Medical Practice 1978* (Chicago, 1978), p. 147.

a physician is classified as hospital-based only if he is employed by a hospital for the largest proportion of his hours of work. Thus, for example, a U.S. radiologist who spends almost all of his time in a hospital, but is not employed by the hospital, is still classified as office-based.[5] If physicians in both countries were classified on the basis of where they deliver most of their services, the distribution between the hospital and office sectors might be more similar. In fact, if hospital chiefs of staff are counted as office-based, then the proportion of office-based physicians in Germany rises to fifty-three percent.

Another very important division within the German profession is between insurance doctors and strictly private physicians. In order to be reimbursed for the care of publicly insured patients, a physician needs a special permit (*Zulassung*) for insurance practice. As explained in chapter 3, admission to practice for the sickness funds was originally very tightly controlled by the funds and was therefore a comparatively rare privilege. Various changes have since opened up access to insurance practice considerably. The Berlin Treaty of 1913 established the right of physician representation on the committees that granted permits. Later agreements raised the physician/population ratio used by the committees to control the size of fund panels. And finally, in 1960, a decision of the Supreme Constitutional Court declared that any limitation on the total number of insurance doctors was an unconstitutional hinderance to the practice of one's profession. The decision was the result of a complaint brought by the Hartmannbund and the Association of Salaried Physicians, most of whose members worked for hospitals or public agencies.[6]

Permits for insurance practice are granted by *Land*-level committees composed of equal numbers of insurance doctors and fund representatives. Any physician who chooses to see publicly insured patients can obtain a permit as long as he meets certain conditions. He must be licensed, must participate in a six-month internship in an office practice, and must become a member of the AID in his *Land*. A permit for insurance practice is very much like a taxicab medallion. It resembles a property right more than a license to practice. Each permit is valid for a particular "seat" (location) and a particular specialty, and may have other special conditions attached. For example, relatives of a permit holder may be given preference in taking over the seat should it be vacated.[7] In practice, the process of obtaining a permit is pro forma, and a physician can virtually create a new "seat" by listing a new office address. But the formal rules retain a very corporatist flavor and have the potential for becoming a strong regulatory instrument for controlling geographic distribution of physicians.

During the 1970s, there were several efforts to turn the admission system into an instrument to redistribute physicians. One proposal, rejected by Parliament, was that permits be granted only for seats in areas designated as medically underserved in the national health needs plan, and that physicians be allowed to choose their own practice location only when all the designated seats were filled. A weaker planning system was passed in 1976. The AIDs are now responsible for using "all suitable measures" to provide care in underserved areas. If such measures fail, the admissions committees may stop granting permits in overserved areas, but only after all other appropriate measures have been tried.

The vast majority of office-based physicians now participate in the public insurance scheme. Until 1976, a physician could choose to see only patients of the substitute funds or to see patients of all funds. In 1971, 7.9 percent of office-based physicians saw only private patients, 3.3 percent saw private and substitute fund patients, and 88.8 percent saw private, substitute fund, and RVO fund patients.[9] These national figures mask very different patterns of participation on the local level, however. In the North Rhine region in 1972, the proportion of insurance physicians who would accept only substitute fund patients varied between nearly 20 percent and 0.6 percent in different cities.[10]

The separation of the medical profession into distinct sectors creates important political divisions within the profession. The sectors typically have their own interest organizations (see table 4.4), much of whose political activity is concerned with defending or expanding boundaries of their respective sectors. The organizations are constantly engaged in legal disputes about exactly which medical tasks and which patient groups "belong" to each sector. The most successful sector has certainly been the office-based insurance doctors, represented by the AIDs. Once they were chartered as bodies of public law and given a mandate to assure the care of insured persons, they were in a strong position to capture new markets for themselves whenever the legislature mandated broader benefits in compulsory insurance. Particularly when the benefits were in the nature of preventive medicine, conflicts ensued over whether the service should be provided by independent, office-based insurance doctors, or by salaried physicians in the public health agencies.[11]

This "capturing" of a monopoly on new markets has happened

Table 4.4 Voluntary Associations of Physicians

Verband der Ärzte Deutschlands (Hartmannbund)
  association of all physicians for protection of their economic interests
Verband der niedergelassene Ärzte Deutschlands, e. V.
  association of office-based physicians
Verband der angestellten Ärzte Deutschlands (Marburger Bund)
  association of salaried hospital physicians
Verband der leitenden Krankenhausärzte Deutschlands
  association of chiefs of staff
Deutsche Kassenarztverband
  association of insurance doctors (voluntary)
Bund der Deutschen Medizinalbeamten
  association of civil service physicians
Berufsverband der praktischen Ärzte Deutschlands
  association of general practitioners
Verband der Fachärzte Deutschlands
  association of specialists

---

several times since the creation of the insurance doctors' associations. When a maternal and child health program was instituted as a mandatory health insurance benefit, the office-based insurance doctors won the exclusive right to perform the prenatal and well-baby exams. In 1971, the government introduced cancer detection examinations for adults as a mandatory benefit of compulsory insurance, and again the office-based insurance doctors won the exclusive rights to perform these examinations. In 1975 the AIDs challenged the right of sickness funds to reimburse hospitals for the preventive examinations performed on newborn infants, and the court upheld the argument of the AIDs that the sickness funds could not contract with hospitals to perform these examinations.[12] This particular challenge, and the court's willingness to support the AIDs, would seem to create additional pressure for hospitals to grant staff privileges to office-based pediatricians.

Specialization. Like the American medical profession, the West German profession is divided into different specialties. As with other structural characteristics, however, specialization does not have quite the same meaning in the two countries. In the United States, formal specialty certifications are granted by nationwide specialty boards for each specialty. The boards conduct formal

Table 4.5 Specialization of Physicians in West Germany and United States

Year	West Germany		United States	
	Number of Non-Specialists*	Non-Specialists as % of All Active Physicians	Number of General Practitioners	General Practitioners as % of All Active Physicians
1963	47,305	57.0	73,055	27.9
1964	48,536	57.6	71,935	26.6
1965	49,222	57.4	70,788	25.5
1966	49,010	56.5	69,611	24.3
1967	49,914	56.4	68,306	23.2
1968	51,078	56.2	60,296	20.3
1969	53,358	56.8	57,845	19.0
1970	58,007	58.2	56,926	18.3
1971	60,257	60.2	55,284	17.3
1972	61,955	57.7	54,558	17.0
1973	63,392	57.1	52,918	16.3
1974	64,137	55.9	53,152	16.3
1975	64,627	54.4	54,557	16.0
1976	65,820	53.9	54,332	15.9
1977	66,504	53.1	55,724	13.1

Note: *For West Germany, these figures include "Fachärzte für Allgemein Medizin," a specialty comparable to family practice in the U.S., as well as all specialists in training.
Sources: Statistisches Bundesamt, *Statistisches Jahrbuch für die Bundesrepublik Deutschland*, annual volumes; American Medical Association, Center for Health Services Research and Development, *Distribution of Physicians in the U.S.*, annual volumes.

examinations, and a certification is valid for the entire country. However, any physician may call himself a specialist and provide specialty services to his patients, without a formal certification. In West Germany, a physician may not call himself a specialist or provide specialty services to his patients without a specialty certification. Certifications for all specialties are granted by a single specialty committee of each chamber of physicians. The committees set educational standards for specialization, but there is no formal examination. Specialty certification is valid for the entire country.[13]

The degree of specialization in the two countries is difficult to compare, since West German statistics group general practitioners, family physicians, and specialists-in-training into one category (tables 4.5 and 4.6). However, given the figures in table 4.5, it is probably safe to say that specialization is less prevalent in West Germany and increasing less rapidly than in the United States.

The most important difference between specialists in the two countries lies in their ability simultaneously to conduct a general practice. In the United States, a specialist is free to provide general services for patients, in addition to the services of his own specialty. And since a formal board certification is not necessary to call oneself a specialist in the United States, American physicians can legally provide any services that fall within the scope of medical practice. In West Germany, specialist physicians are specifically prohibited by the Federal Physicians' Code from practicing general medicine. A specialist "may not develop his practice into a general primary care practice; he may not separate his patients from their own general practitioner."[14] One implication of this difference in the legal rights of American and West German specialists is that the comparative statistics show more of a difference than really exists. Since American specialists can and do provide general services, the availability of general services in the United States is higher than the statistics based on specialty designations would indicate.

The difference in the legal rights of specialists probably ex-

Table 4.6 Specialization of West German Physicians by Sector, 1976

Sector	All Physicians	Office-Based	Hospital Chiefs of Staff	Other Hospital-Based	Administrative
Specialists	49,025	25,346	6,653	14,038	2,988
	(45.1%)	(49.7%)	(94.3%)	(32.2%)	(42.9%)
Nonspecialists*	59,665	25,669	405	29,621	3,970
	(54.9%)	(50.3%)	(5.7%)	(67.8%)	(57.1%)
Total	108,690	51,015	7,058	43,659	6,958
	(100%)	(100%)	(100%)	(100%)	(100%)

Note: *Includes specialists in general medicine, as well as all specialists in training.
Source: Klaus Gehb, "Die ärztliche Versorgung in der Bundesrepublik Deutschland: Ergebnisse der Ärztestatistik zum l. Januar 1976," Deutsches Ärzteblatt (1976), table 3. There are some small discrepancies between the subtotals and the totals in Gehb's table. Only Gehb's subtotals were used. The absolute figures may not be entirely accurate, but the relative proportions should be reasonably accurate.

plains much of the lower degree of specialization in West Germany. In the United States, a person who declares himself a specialist or who obtains formal specialty certification is not forced to derive his entire income from the practice of his specialty. In choosing a specialty, he does not need to worry whether there is a big enough market for his services, because he can provide any mix of specialty and generalist services for which he has patient demand. And he can practice general medicine while he gradually builds a practice in his specialty. Specialization is thus not economically risky for the American physician, yet it can provide him with a competitive advantage in that he can distinguish his services from those of other physicians. For the West German physician, specialization represents a definite economic risk, because it narrows the range of services the physician can provide. For office-based specialists, the range of services is further restricted by the lack of staff privileges.

The West German system of specialization is another vestige of the corporatist tradition, in which the work of different occupations was rigidly divided and tightly controlled by occupational chambers. Like the other sector divisions in West German medicine, the specialty divisions are designed to prevent competition among the different professional subgroups and to preserve the security of each group. Ironically, though, the West German system forces physicians to consider the market demand for their services when they choose whether and how to specialize. The comparison of the two countries suggests that if similar restrictions were introduced in the United States, and physicians were forced to be more responsive to market forces in their professional career choices, the United States might begin to have more general practitioners.

Organization of Office-Based Practices. As in the United States, the political organizations of the medical profession have sought to protect the solo practitioner from competition with clinics by preventing the development of group practices. In West Germany, physicians must receive permission from their chamber to form a group practice. The chambers have strongly opposed group practices and have prohibited them through provisions of the Federal Physicians' Code. In 1968, the umbrella organization of state chambers, the Federal Chamber of Physicians (BÄK), liberalized its policy on group practices, but it still opposes the formation of multispecialty groups.[15] Since professional interaction and referral among different specialists within a single group is seen by physicians as a major advantage of group practice, the BÄK's policy is still a significant hindrance to the formation of group practices. The physicians' code also states that a group practice must meet the desire of patients who wish to be seen by a single physician. This requirement nullifies a major advantage of group practices—the ability of the individual physician to control his working hours by sharing patients with a group of colleagues. As a result of these restrictions, there are very few group practices in West Germany.[16]

West German physicians also require the permission of their chambers to add paramedical personnel and to hire a temporary replacement while they go on vacation.[17] The use of ancillary personnel in offices is apparently greater in West Germany than in the United States. In 1971, the average personnel per office (including the physician) was 4.6 in West Germany and 2.5 to 3.0 in the United States.[18] Between 1963 and 1971, the average office size in West Germany grew nearly 25 percent (from 3.7 to 4.6 people per practice).[19] Since a physician can be reimbursed for procedures performed by ancillary personnel, the chambers have no reason to oppose expanded use of assistants.

As part of their general effort to prevent competition among physicians, the chambers also limit office hours.[20] In public discussions about the enormous increase in volume of physicians' services in the last several years, physicians have vehemently argued that the "productivity" increases are due to increases in physicians' working hours. The sickness funds, on the other hand, report that physicians' announced office hours have continually declined.[21] These claims are difficult to substantiate, since there do not seem to be any systematic surveys of physicians' practices as there are in the United States.

One aspect of the organization of office practices that is not regulated is capital investment. It has long been part of the conventional wisdom of West German health policy analysts that the acquisition of machines (particularly laboratory apparatus and radiation equipment) by office practitioners is the major cause of the tremendous growth in volume of services. Here, too, there is a dearth of empirical data, but the few empirical studies suggest that investment in capital equipment is quite low: in 1971, the total value of new purchases and depreciation of old equipment comprised only 3.1 percent of the gross income of the average practice and less than 10 percent of the costs of a practice.[22]

In summary, there are several important differences between

the West German and American medical professions which the American reader should keep in mind. Most importantly, the West German medical profession is divided into sectors of practice whose boundaries may not be crossed by individual physicians, except to change "careers." Except for about ten percent of office-based physicians and about six percent of hospital-based physicians, physicians in either sector cannot deliver care in the other. In order to be reimbursed for ambulatory services to patients in the public health insurance scheme, office-based physicians must obtain a special permit, and no other physicians (such as hospital physicians or public health service doctors) may be reimbursed through the scheme. The vast majority (about eighty-eight percent) of office-based doctors do participate in the scheme. West Germany has a higher physician/population ratio than the United States, and a much higher proportion of nonspecialists in both the ambulatory and hospital sectors. Specialists in West Germany are restricted to practicing their particular specialties. And finally, some aspects of the internal organization of office practices are regulated more stringently than in the United States—notably, the formation of group practices.

Allocative Decisions of Individual Physicians

Medical services, unlike many commodities and services, are generally purchased on the advice of a technical expert. Any decision to purchase medical care, beyond an initial visit to a physician, is strongly influenced by the advice of a physician. Many services, especially hospital care, some specialist care, and prescription drugs, can be purchased *only* with the permission of a physician. The combination of the imbalance in technical knowledge between physicians and patients, professional referral patterns, and legal restrictions on the purchase of drugs puts the physician in a central position in the determination of demand for medical services. Not surprisingly, then, economists have found that the supply of physicians in a given area is a major determinant of the demand for medical services.[23] Similarly, in the hospital sector, it has been found that the supply of beds in a given area is an important determinant of the actual rate of hospitalization there.[24]

In West Germany, there is considerable evidence that ambulatory care physicians are able to expand the volume of "necessary" services very readily. At times when large numbers of new physicians have been admitted to insurance practice, the volume of services billed to sickness funds has grown in virtually the same proportion as the increase in number of physicians.[25] Sickness funds have found an inverse relationship between the number of cases in a physician's practice and the number of procedures performed per case, suggesting that physicians aim for a target income, and manipulate the number of procedures as their caseload changes.[26]

In a system of nearly universal public health insurance with comprehensive benefits, physicians acquire enormous control over the expenditure of significant amounts of public funds. Because patients essentially delegate their consumption decisions to physicians, and because a health insurance program entitles patients to receive whatever care a physician deems necessary, physicians effectively become the "authorized purchasing agent" of health services. Their medical decisions are simultaneously a recommendation to the patient about what services to buy, and an authorization from the government to pay for the same services. Not surprisingly, then, sickness fund managers as well as government officials look on doctors as the key to expenditure control. More specifically, office-based doctors are seen as the gatekeepers for the three major components of sickness fund expenditures—ambulatory services, hospital services, and prescription drugs.

Approximately eighteen percent of sickness fund expenditures go directly for the services of office-based physicians. Public health insurance covers all diagnostic and therapeutic services performed by a physician or physician's assistant[27] in an office. Consultations, home visits, examinations, and diagnostic and therapeutic procedures done in an office are all covered. There is no cost sharing by patients (for example, coinsurance or deductibles) for either in-hospital or outpatient care. Doctors are considered to have nearly complete freedom to determine what services and procedures they perform, given that they have been engaged by the patient. They retain a large amount of discretion in deciding what diagnostic tests to order, how to treat the problems that are presented to them, and when to refer to (more expensive) specialists.

To some (perhaps very large) extent, physicians' decisions about diagnostic and therapeutic services are constrained by the frequency and types of injuries and illness presented to them. But illness is not a totally objective concept that exists apart from physicians' willingness to label problems as illness. Physicians also have a great deal of discretion in deciding whether to treat a patient's complaints as symptomatic of a medical problem requiring treatment, a personal problem requiring either counseling or no treatment at all, or a strategic attempt by the patient to obtain some secondary benefit (such as a sick leave certificate, a prescription drug, or a legitimate excuse for not doing something unpleasant).[28] Thus, physicians also exercise some indirect control on the volume of health expenditures in that they help to define the level of medical illness in a population.

Another major category of sickness fund expenditures, accounting for approximately thirty percent, is hospital care. Virtually all hospital care is covered by social health insurance, if recommended by an office-based physician or required in an emergency. Until 1974, coverage included a maximum of 72 weeks in a hospital for any one illness within two years, but as of 1974 unlimited time in a hospital has been covered. Office-based physicians have some control over the cost of in-hospital services. Since all patients require a referral by an office doctor to be treated in a hospital (except in emergencies), the number of referrals authorized by the panel doctors directly affects the costs to a sickness fund for specialist and hospital services.

Prescription drugs and medical appliances account for about nineteen percent of sickness fund expenditures. All prescription drugs and medical appliances (e.g., glasses, corsets, arch supports, baths, physical therapy) are covered by social insurance, but with a coinsurance rate of twenty percent, up to a maximum of DM 1 (less than $1.00). Since these can be obtained only with a doctor's prescription, doctors are seen as responsible for the volume of expenditures on drugs and appliances. The cost to a sickness fund for prescription drugs is directly a function of the number and cost (price) of prescriptions written by physicians in its panel.

In addition to their influence over the volume of physicians' services, hospital services, and prescription items, physicians in West Germany have some control over another very expensive resource: human labor. Health insurance in Germany has always included some form of wage continuation payments for workers; some of the cash benefits were paid by the sickness funds, and some by employers, but cash benefits have been a major expense of the health insurance system.

Until 1966, cash benefits constituted the single largest expenditure of the sickness funds. (Cash benefits include some other benefits in addition to wage continuation payments, but the wage continuation payments are the most important component.) In the period from 1957 to 1962, when health insurance reform and cost control were major national issues, cash benefits accounted for more than twenty-seven percent of sickness fund expenditures. The new wage continuation law of 1970, requiring employers, rather than sickness funds, to cover the first six weeks of wage continuation payments to their employees, has had the effect of drastically reducing sickness fund expenditures on cash benefits to less than ten percent of total expenditures.

Wage continuation payments, because they were a major expenditure of sickness funds, were also the cause for one of the distinctive institutions of the health insurance scheme, the "sick leave certificate." In order for a person to collect wage continuation payments, he must be certified as "unable to work" by an insurance doctor. Physicians thus not only legitimize absenteeism in a moral sense, but also make official decisions about eligibility for a major income replacement program. Thus, office-based physicians, through their decisions to issue sick leave certificates, influence the volume of wage continuation payments, and to some extent the level of absenteeism in the work force.

To the extent that physician availability influences consumer use of services, the decisions of individual physicians about whether to participate in government programs can have a strong impact on the success of government efforts to alter patterns of medical care. The government's preventive care program is a good example. In July 1971, the government introduced a preventive care program that required all sickness funds to offer cancer screening examinations for women over thirty and men over forty-five, as well as a series of seven general preventive examinations for children under five.[29] Guidelines published by the Ministry of Labor prescribe specific procedures and tests that are to be performed for each type of examination. The cost of the examinations is covered in the regular insurance premiums, although the insured must obtain a (free) special entitlement coupon from the sickness fund.

Participation in the program during the first year was low. Approximately twenty percent of eligible women, nine percent of eligible men, and forty percent of eligible children took advantage of the program.[30] An evaluation study conducted by the Ministry of Labor found significant differences in utilization rates by age, type of sickness fund, and type of information received by the insured about the program. Most notably, when the sickness fund mailed an entitlement coupon along with its individual

Table 4.7 Physician Participation in Preventive Screening Program, First Quarter of 1972

Type of Examination	Type of Physician						
	Family Practice	Surgery	Derma-tology	Internal Medicine	Urology	Gyne-cology	Pediat-rics
Male cancer screening	65.34%	61.92%	40.78%	72.87%	98.93%		
Female cancer screening	41.29	14.76				100.33%	
Well-baby exams	48.61			6.40		38.50	99.42%

Note: These figures include noninsurance doctors who participate (under a special provision in this program), although the base used as 100% includes only licensed insurance doctors. Thus, the participation rates among insurance doctors in these specialties are actually lower. Another problem is that participation was measured by whether each doctor had collected an entitlement coupon—i.e., whether an examination was actually performed. This means that physicians who were willing to perform an exam but had no patient requests were not counted.
Source: Deutscher Bundestag, 7. Wahlperiode, Drucksache 7/454, "Bericht der Bundesregierung über die Erfahrung mit der Einführung von Maßnahmen zur Früherkennung von Krankheiten," table 2, pp. 16–19.

mailing of program information, participation increased to thirty-five percent among women and nearly sixteen percent among men.[31]

Rates of participation by different kinds of physicians were widely divergent, as table 4.7 shows. There was also a wide variation in participation rates among physicians in different localities. For example, among family practitioners in the well-baby examinations rates varied from 11.3 percent in Berlin to 68.7 percent in Schleswig-Holstein. Although the study does not provide enough data to correlate patient utilization rates with physician participation rates, it seems highly probable that physicians' willingness to participate in the program and their readiness to recommend the examinations to their patients have a significant impact on patient utilization rates. The director of a large municipal sickness fund said he believes that many physicians do not do the full screening examinations because they can be reimbursed more for performing some of the procedures separately and billing under the regular fee schedule.[32] Although the evidence is not yet in, it seems likely that West German physicians have a significant impact on the volume of preventive screening provided.

It is clear that physicians as individuals have considerable authority in the implementation of a public health insurance program. Beyond their role as advisers to patients, they inevitably become allocators of the benefits. In West Germany, physicians preside not only over the distribution of medical goods and services, but also over an enormous cash transfer program for temporarily disabled workers.

The discretionary power of physicians derives from a combination of several elements: the technical ability of physicians actually to cure or improve some problems; the cultural belief that certain kinds of problems can be helped by physicians; legal requirements that grant physicians exclusive rights to perform certain kinds of activities; and the persuasive abilities of individual physicians. But ultimately, the types of discretionary authority we have examined in this chapter derive from the collective power of the profession, because it is the public policymaking process, not the individual consultation, that sets the structure within which physicians conduct their medical practice.

Once a government assumes some responsibility for the allocation of health care resources, it faces the central problem of deciding exactly how to do so. How much health care should it require or encourage people to buy, and what limits, if any, should it impose on their health care purchases? The problem is under-scored by the highly technical nature of much medical care and the dual role of physicians as both expert advisers on the kind and amount of care necessary and suppliers of most medical goods and services. But as a matter of public policy, the issue is not merely to decide on the technical criteria for the allocation of health care resources, but also to establish structures of decisionmaking that will result in the desired behavior of patients and physicians.

Societies have many choices in establishing these decision-making structures. A government can attempt to regulate the allocative decisions of physicians directly. It can also regulate the more fundamental career decisions and choices about the structure of practice which influence the allocative decisions. West Germany regulates these fundamental decisions more closely than does the United States. But on the whole, these second order choices are not very heavily regulated in either West Germany or the United States, when contrasted with other countries with more centralized systems, such as Great Britain, Sweden, the Soviet Union, or the People's Republic of China. These countries represent another range of political choices in the regulation of physicians, in which many of the decisions about entering the medical profession, choosing a specialty, and locat-ing and organizing a practice are even more directly controlled by government.

Chapters 5 through 8 examine some mechanisms in the West German health system that are aimed more directly at the allocative authority of physicians—that is, the power of physi-cians to determine the expenditure of public funds. The mecha-nisms are structural features of the health system which are the result of deliberate policy choices. While the collective power of the medical profession was certainly important in the formation of these policy decisions, the decisions were in no way determined by the technical nature of medical care. The four mechanisms to be studied are the creation by the federal government of large countervailing organizations of health care consumers and pro-viders; the method of reimbursing physicians; the system of government mandated peer review of office-based physicians, known as economic monitoring; and the separate system of peer review to monitor the sick leave certificates granted by office-based physicians.

Chapter Five | Limits on Collective Power: Countervailing Organizations

The Strategy of Countervailing Power

One of the most notable features of the German health insurance system is the corporatization of authority. Individual patients and physicians have no authority to negotiate about fees and payments. They confront each other in the office as individuals with equal power (or lack of power) to influence the economic behavior of the other. Physicians and patients meet each other not as individual buyers and sellers in a market, but rather as members of large organizations that engage in collective bargaining.

The strategy of countervailing power has been discussed at length by John Kenneth Galbraith. In *American Capitalism*, he argues that the concentration of sellers into a few oligopolistic firms often stimulates a parallel concentration of buyers into large countervailing organizations.[1] Collective organization may sometimes be accomplished without the coercive power of the state, but often groups seek and require state support in order to organize effectively. In Galbraith's view, one of the key functions of government is to control conflict by balancing competing interests. Although the validity of Galbraith's theory as an empirical description of the American economy and government has been widely criticized,[2] it provides a useful framework for analyzing the development of German health policy.

The parallel evolution of physicians' and patients' organizations is striking. Sickness funds were originally voluntary associations of workers, mainly for the purpose of protecting themselves against income loss during illness. The funds themselves had some role in procuring medical services for their members but served primarily as savings or insurance institutions. Professional scientific associations of physicians, as well as professional political organizations such as the Leipziger Verband, were also originally voluntary membership organizations with no official authority to govern the conduct of either members or nonmembers. The introduction of compulsory health insurance in 1883 required the participating sickness funds to offer medical service benefits as well as income replacement benefits. Numerous voluntary or private welfare funds (*Freie Hilfskassen*) also began to offer medical service benefits under competitive pressure from the statutory sickness funds. Physicians found themselves having to deal more and more with these funds as organized representatives of groups of patients, rather than with individual patients, in order to have access to a large patient market. The political and economic strength of the sickness funds gave impetus to physicians to organize themselves, and eventually to bargain with sickness funds only on a collective basis. The sickness funds in turn organized themselves into large voluntary interest associations (see chapter 3 above).

It has been argued that development of large countervailing compulsory membership organizations proceeded according to an almost inevitable internal dynamic.[3] In this interpretation, the development of sickness funds was the response of consumers to the monopolistic control exercised by physicians. At a later stage, the development of large medical-political organizations was the response of physicians to the dominant position of the then highly organized consumers. And the consolidation of funds was their response to physician organization.

But it would be a mistake to see the development of large corporative organizations as the product of some natural evolutionary process. Just as liberal market societies could not evolve without a series of government decisions to support the formation of markets,[4] the corporatist form of organization in Germany could not have evolved without the support of certain deliberate political decisions. Early decisions by the various German states and principalities created the regulatory structure of chamber self-government and granted chamber status to physicians. The decision to create national health insurance as a service benefit program administered through independent sickness funds further shaped the relationships among physicians, patients, employers, insurers, and government agencies. And finally, the series of central government decrees in the years between 1923 and 1932 created the modern system of collective bargaining between sickness funds and associations of insurance doctors. Clearly, both consumer and provider organizations had begun to form *before* the government mandated their existence; the government certainly did not create them out of whole cloth. But government policy certainly accelerated their development and increased their power by investing them with quasi-governmental authority.

To evaluate the effectiveness of the countervailing power strategy, one needs to ask, first, to what extent the government (and consumers) succeeded in creating large organizations capable of acting as a strong, unified force; second, how well these organizations function as consumer membership organizations; third, how equitably the sickness funds distribute the costs of health services; and finally, whether they succeed in procuring medical services at lower cost than individuals or smaller groups might be able to obtain.

The Organization of Sickness Funds

The contemporary health insurance program is administered by about fourteen hundred separate sickness funds, whose membership structure reflects the corporatist origins of the system. The categories of sickness funds are defined primarily by the broad occupational status of their members. The RVO funds were created by the national health insurance program. They are primarily for compulsorily insured people, although they also include voluntary members. Within this RVO category, there are four types of funds: factory funds (*Betriebskrankenkassen*), for employees of enterprises large enough to have at least 450 employees subject to compulsory insurance; guild funds (*Innungskrankenkassen*), for people in trades, crafts, and services, such as barbers, bakers, shoemakers, or plumbers; agricultural funds (*Landwirtschaftliche Krankenkassen*), organized on a geographic basis and covering people in the agricultural sector; and local funds (*Ortskrankenkassen*), also organized on a geographic basis and covering all workers who do not come under the jurisdiction of other funds. Two occupations have entirely separate funds—miners (*Bundesknappschaft*) and mariners (*Seekasse*). The special status of these groups probably derives from their historical position as the most strongly organized occupations during the period from about 1900 to 1920 when the insurance system was created and assumed its basic character.

Additionally, there is a separate group of holdover or "substitute funds" (*Ersatzkassen*) which existed as mutual aid societies before national health insurance came into effect. They have been allowed to persist, but no new ones may be formed. The substitute funds must accept as members any person for whom insurance is compulsory, who lives in their geographic jurisdiction, and who fits into the occupational category they cover. These funds are regulated much like the RVO funds, and may not refuse to accept a person because of age or health status. Finally, there are private insurance companies which are not part of the national health insurance system.

In 1977, there was a total of 1,396 funds, of which 301 were local, 901 were factory funds, 158 were guild funds, 19 were agricultural, 8 were substitute funds for blue-collar workers, 7 were substitute funds for white-collar workers, one was a miners' and one a seamen's fund. The local sickness funds are most important in that they provide coverage for nearly half of all insured persons. In the past twenty years, substitute funds for white-collar workers have gained an increasing share of the insurance market and now cover well over one-quarter of the population (see table 5.1).

One prerequisite for an effective countervailing power strategy is that large organizations of consumers must actually be created. An indicator of successful organizational growth of the sickness funds is the proportion of the population enrolled. Statutory

Table 5.1 Percentage of All Insured Persons Covered by the Various Kinds of Sickness Funds

| Year | Local | Agri-cultural | Fac-tory | Guild | Miners | Sea-men | Substitute | |
							White-Collar	Blue-Collar
1955	61.5	2.4	13.0	2.9	5.9	0.2	13.2	0.6
1960	57.0	1.7	13.3	3.5	5.2	0.3	18.2	0.9
1965	53.7	1.5	13.5	4.3	4.6	0.3	21.2	1.0
1970	52.3	1.4	13.6	4.6	3.7	0.3	23.0	1.1
1975	48.2	2.8	12.7	4.7	3.2	0.2	27.4	1.1
1977	48.0	2.7	12.5	4.8	3.1	0.2	27.5	1.1

Sources: 1955–70: *Statistiches Jahrbuch der Kassenärztlichen Bundesvereinigung*, 1971, p. 12. 1975–77: Bundesministerium für Arbeit und Sozialordnung, "Statistiche Daten zur konzertierten Aktion im Gesundheitswesen," 28 February 1978, table 3.

Table 5.2 Categorical Expansion of Health Insurance

1883 Blue-collar workers
1903 Transport and commercial (office) workers
1911 Agricultural and forestry workers, domestic servants
1914 Civil Service employees
1918 Unemployed
1927 Seamen
1930 Dependents of fund members
1941 Voluntary public insurance (workers no longer eligible for compulsory insurance owing to wage increases that put their income over the ceiling could now elect to continue their coverage with the same fund voluntarily)
1941 Pensioners
1966 Farmworkers (*Landarbeiter*) and salesmen (*Händler*)
1972 Self-employed agricultural workers and dependents
1975 Students and handicapped persons

Sources: Compiled from Christa Altenstetter, "Urban Decision-Making in Federal Systems: A Comparative Analysis of the Delivery System of Health Services in the United States and West Germany," Urban Institute, unpublished monograph, June 30, 1972); and Bundesministerium für Arbeit und Sozialordnung, *Übersicht über die Soziale Sicherung*, 1970, pp. 121–22, and 1977, p. 184.

health insurance has gradually absorbed an increasing share of the population, until now over ninety percent of the population is insured through the scheme. Most of the expansion in coverage occurred through successive legislative reforms to include more social categories of people in the compulsory insurance program (see table 5.2).

Another measure of organizational strength is the degree of concentration of the sickness funds. While the number of fund participants was increasing, both absolutely and as a proportion of the total population, the number of sickness funds was actually declining, and the average fund size growing larger (see table 5.3). This pattern of consolidation of funds means that physicians over time have had to bargain with increasingly larger organizations that represent an increasing proportion of patients.

Nevertheless, there are two important factors that tend to weaken the ability of the funds to act as a large unified representative of consumer interests. First, there is a substantial market for health services outside the public health insurance system. Exactly how large this market is cannot be determined, because the government does not collect any data on private sector health insurance or health services payments. A report of the Ministry of Health estimated that in 1968 only about fifty-two percent of all expenditures for health services were from the statutory sickness funds.[5] But this is a very rough estimate, by the ministry's own admission, and West German analysts are reluctant to give very much credit to this guess. A study conducted by an American

Table 5.3 Consolidation of Sickness Funds

Year	Number of Funds	Average Number of Full Members per Fund
1911	22,000	455
1914	13,500	1,185
1932	6,600	2,833
1938	4,600	5,044
1951	1,992	10,040
1955	2,070	10,966
1960	2,028	13,363
1965	1,972	14,554
1970	1,827	16,749
1973	1,627	20,405
1976	1,425	23,509

Source: Calculated from Bundesministerium für Arbeit und Sozialordnung, *Übersicht über die Soziale Sicherung*, 1975, p. 153, and 1977, p. 181.

research firm estimates that 10.6 million people (or about one-sixth of the population) carry private insurance. Of these, 4.4 million carry private insurance exclusively and 6.2 million carry supplementary private insurance. The same study estimated that private health expenditures in 1976, not including wage continuation payments, were about DM 5 billion, as compared with expenditures of DM 57.8 billion by the statutory health insurance programs.[6] Still another indicator of the size of the private sector is the proportion of physicians' income that derives from private practice. Currently, the Ministry of Labor estimates this figure at about fifteen percent.[7] While this represents a sizeable proportion of services, the size of physicians' private practice seems to have been declining over time (see table 5.4), indicating that the public funds have been able to control a growing proportion of expenditures, at least for physician services.

The second weakness of the sickness funds—and one that receives the most attention in West German policy discussions—is competition between the substitute funds and RVO funds within the statutory health insurance system. The substitute funds, though regulated as part of the public insurance scheme, have always retained more prestige than the RVO funds and are seen as something between statutory and private insurance. In order to compete with private insurance, they offer broader coverage to their members and pay higher fees to physicians than the RVO funds provide. The RVO funds are then pressured to offer similar benefits in order not to be accused of providing "second class care."[8] One aspect of this dynamic is that the benefits offered by the substitute funds slowly become part of the customary standard of care. The RVO funds are also under pressure to match

Table 5.4 Proportion of Total Income of Office-Based Physicians Derived from Private Practice

Year	Percent
1950	30.2%
1954	27.0
1959	23.5
1963	22.1
1965	20.0
1971	15.0

Sources: 1950–65: Josef Stockhausen, *Deutsches Ärzteblatt* (1965), cited by Paul Lüth, *Niederlassung und Praxis* (Stuttgart: Georg Thieme, 1969), p. 96. 1971: Bundesministerium für Arbeit und Sozialordnung, *Übersicht über die Soziale Sicherung,* 1975, p. 166.

the fees of the substitute funds, because of the popular belief that when a physician is paid more he provides higher quality services.

The precise impact of the competition between the RVO funds and the substitute funds is difficult to determine, but it is clear that such competition exists. RVO fund administrators point to advertisements by the substitute funds in which vacations at spas are offered to prospective members as an inducement to join,[9] and to evidence that they are more liberal in granting spa treatments as medically necessary[10] and in allowing prescription items.[11]

Technically, the substitute funds are not allowed to use illness risk factors in selecting their members.[12] But an examination of membership figures for the different types of funds (see table 5.5) suggests that the substitute funds are indeed very successful at "cream-skimming," that is, selecting the better risks. The substitute funds insure 33.4 percent of all fund members, but only 14.5 percent of pensioners (who can be expected to require more than average medical services). Moreover, the substitute funds insure 66 percent of all voluntary members, who are primarily white-collar workers with relatively higher incomes (i.e., incomes above the minimum for compulsory membership), and who therefore can be expected to be relatively low-risk members. That the substitute funds compete with private insurance for voluntary members is suggested by the fact that over thirty percent of substitute fund members are voluntary. By contrast, only about 5 percent of the local fund members are volunatry.[13]

The skewed distribution of risks portrayed in table 5.5 suggests

Table 5.5 Distribution of Members and Expenditures among Fund Types, 1974

	Type of Fund				
Distribution	Local	Factory	Guild	Agri-cultural	Substi-tute
All members[a]	45.2%	13.4%	5.6%	2.4%	33.4%
All pensioners[a]	64.7	13.6	2.7	4.5	14.5
All voluntary members[b]	20.7	7.8	3.3		66.9
All expenditures[a]	50.2	13.9	4.4	2.8	29.11

Sources: [a] Theo Siebeck, *Zur Kostenentwicklung in der Krankenversicherung* (Bonn: Bundesverband der Ortskrankenkassen, 1976) pp. 123–25. [b] Bundesverband der Ortskrankenkassen, "Statistischer Vierteljahresbericht: Die Ortskrankenkassen im Jahre 1977" (Bonn, 1978), table 3. These figures do not include agricultural funds.

that the public health insurance system has not been completely successful in creating a strong, unified organization of health care consumers. Despite the incorporation of the preexisting sickness funds (substitute funds) into the public insurance scheme, and despite efforts to subject them to the same requirements as the RVO funds, they have managed to retain a quasi-private character and to select out better risks for their membership and offer greater benefits than the RVO funds.

Internal Government of the Sickness Funds

In assessing the efficacy of sickness funds as representatives of consumer interests in the health care sector, it is important to know how well the funds actually articulate the interests of their members. Since the funds are formally institutions of self-management, an examination of their internal governing structures will shed some light on the extent of consumer influence on their policies.

The government of the sickness funds is described by the by-laws of each fund. The by-laws set out the structure of internal government, the criteria for membership, and the level of benefits. In fact, most of these features are to a large degree fixed by the Imperial Insurance Code, so there is little difference between various funds. All funds are governed by a representative assembly composed of equal numbers of employees' and employers' representatives. Employees' representatives are chosen in elections run by the trade unions; employers' representatives are chosen by the employers' unions. This assembly, whose size is limited by law to a maximum of sixty members, elects an executive committee usually with about ten to fifteen members.

Representation on these governing bodies is based on contributions to the insurance scheme. Since employers and employees pay matching contributions to the scheme, each group is entitled to fifty percent of the votes in internal government. However, family members, who comprise about forty percent of insured persons, have no direct representation, and voluntary members, who until 1971 paid their entire premium without an employer contribution, did not have a correspondingly stronger voice in the assembly. In the substitute funds, employers have no representation in the representative assemblies, and in the miners' fund, employers have only one-third representation.[14]

The role of the representative assembly is primarily to establish the by-laws of the fund and to elect the executive committee. The assembly must also ratify the budget, vote on any supplementary benefits to be offered in addition to compulsory benefits, and set the exact rate for contributions. Positions on both the representative assembly and the executive committee are honorary and unpaid. The executive committee elects a director or board of directors, who are professional managers working full time in fund management as their primary occupation. The executive committee is responsible for supervising these directors and ensuring that they carry out the will of the representative assembly, and for representing the fund in any judicial or administrative proceedings. The board of directors makes most of the day-to-day decisions, manages the use of personnel and material resources, and prepares the information and proposals on which the organs of self-administration eventually vote.[15]

As might be expected from the above description, self-administration in practice is quite weak. A survey conducted in 1975 by one of the major public opinion research institutes found general ignorance about and apathy toward self-management in social insurance. Only twenty-seven percent of respondents said they had ever even heard of self-administration in the sickness funds. Eighty-six percent said they would not accept a voluntary position in sickness fund self-government. Forty-three percent felt that social insurance is too technical for lay persons and ought to be administered by specialists. When asked whether they were aware of the social insurance elections held the previous year, only forty percent of respondents said yes. And forty-eight percent believed that participation in social insurance elections is either superfluous or of no concern to them.[16]

One indicator of the professionalization of fund management is the 1971 amendment to the 1969 Law on Occupational Education[17] which made "social insurance administrative specialists" an officially recognized occupation. Under this new law and subsequent administrative regulations, the training of social insurance specialists through schools and apprenticeships with sickness funds was standardized and intensified. Formal guidelines for the length and content of study programs as well as for qualifying examinations were established by the Ministry of Labor.[18]

Another indicator of the weakness of self-management is the low rate of participation in social insurance elections. Surprisingly, little empirical research on participation in these elections has been conducted in West Germany, but a few statistics will serve to illustrate the low rates. In the elections of 1958, voting rates in three substitute funds were reported as 33 percent, 29 percent, and 24 percent. In the 1962 elections, the overall rate of participation was estimated at 25 percent.[19] In 1968, when 52 of approximately 2,100 sickness funds held elections, only 19.3 percent of the eligible voters actually cast ballots.[20] These figures are strikingly low in the context of West German politics, where participation rates in national elections have been consistently greater than 75 percent since 1903 and greater than 85 percent since 1953.[21] Even in state and local elections, between 45 and 60 percent of eligible voters usually vote.[22]

Since norms of electoral participation appear to be very strong in Germany, one must look for some other explanation for the low rates of participation in sickness fund self-government. Several explanations have been advanced by German sociologists. One theory is that the doctor-patient relationship is so much more salient than the relationship between fund members and administrators that members are much more interested in the medical services provided by the funds than in management.[23] A related argument holds that consumers are unaware of the importance of health policy until they have a medical crisis.[24] Another explanation emphasizes the weak and indirect contact between insured persons and their funds. Patients rarely have a need to visit the fund or communicate with fund administrators, since contributions are deducted by employers and not paid directly by the insured, and since the fund pays physicians directly without patients having to submit a bill.[25]

Still another explanation for the lack of participation in fund elections is the perfunctory nature of the elections themselves. (Here it is of course hard to separate cause and effect.) The law on self-administration permits sickness funds to omit elections when there is only one list of candidates. These so-called "peace elections" are apparently predominant except among very large sickness funds.[26]

Finally, perhaps the most important explanation is that national elections are potentially much more effective than social insurance elections for changing the character of the health insurance program. Because the different funds are based primarily on occupational and income categories, the income distribution within any one fund tends to be relatively homogeneous.[27] Even if the members could effect major policy changes within a given fund, the changes would be unlikely to have a significant redistributional impact. On the other hand, social insurance is frequently a major topic of debate between the parties in national election campaigns, and important changes in population coverage, benefit structure, and incidence of tax burden have generally been introduced at the national level (see table 5.6).

Table 5.6 Major Legislative Changes in National Health Insurance Benefits

1883	Medical service benefits and cash benefits limited to combined total of 13 weeks.
1903	Benefit period extended to 26 weeks.
1941	Service benefit and cash benefit coverage periods separated.
1943	Limit on service benefit period removed entirely.
1951	Insured workers' contribution reduced from two-thirds to one-half.
1957	Cash benefits (wage continuation payment) for blue-collar workers increased from 65 percent to 90 percent of regular net earnings. Waiting period for cash benefits for blue-collar workers reduced from three days to two days.
1969	Liability for cash benefits for first six weeks of worker's illness transferred from sickness funds to employers. Bonus payment for nonuse of illness vouchers introduced. Cost-sharing for prescription drugs introduced.
1971	Provision for automatic yearly adjustment of income ceiling for compulsory insurance introduced.
1972	Cancer screening examinations introduced as a mandatory benefit.
1974	Unlimited coverage for hospital care introduced as a mandatory benefit (previously limited to 72 weeks). Bonus payments for nonuse of vouchers eliminated.

The foregoing analysis of fund self-government suggests that consumers' participation in the management of their organizations is not very strong. But the weakness of internal democracy does not necessarily mean that the funds are unable to procure substantial benefits for their members. The strength of the national associations of sickness funds as lobby groups and the bargaining power of the funds vis-à-vis the AIDs are probably more important than internal democracy in securing economic advantages for medical care consumers.

Financing of the Sickness Funds

The individual sickness funds are financially autonomous organizations, although federal law establishes certain guidelines within which they must operate. The most important guidelines specified at the national level are the minimum benefit package and the level of taxable earnings. Within these parameters, each fund is responsible for balancing its income and expenditures, as well as for providing necessary and appropriate care to its members.

The funds must finance their expenditures primarily through employer and employee contributions. There are several exceptions to the method of joint contributions, however.[28] Very low wage earners have their entire premium paid by their employers, for example. Premiums for pensioners have traditionally been paid by the pension insurance authorities, but as of 1977 the government will gradually phase in a system requiring pensioners to pay their own premiums. Students must pay a certain fixed amount (in 1977, DM 25 per month). Agricultural workers pay their own premiums, based on the value of their land and agricultural business income. Direct government subsidy of the sickness funds is limited to a few situations: funds receive a subsidy of DM 20 for each insured student and DM 400 for every woman who receives maternity benefits. The federal government also pays premiums for members of the armed services and retired agricultural workers not otherwise covered. All of these other revenue sources comprise only a very small proportion of the funds' income, and their primary revenue raising capacity remains the tax on earned income.

Federal law sets three important parameters that affect the ability of the sickness funds to raise revenues through the payroll tax. First, the law stipulates a minimum earnings level below which public health insurance is compulsory (*Pflichtgrenze*). This level in essence determines the number of white-collar workers who will be compulsorily insured, but since a large proportion of employees with incomes above the level opt to insure themselves voluntarily in the public system, the total number of fund members is not greatly influenced by this parameter. Second, the federal legislature sets the wage base subject to taxation for social insurance (*Beitragsbemessungsgrenze*). In practice, the wage base has always been set at the same level as the minimum earnings level. Thirdly, until recently, the legislature set a ceiling on the tax rate at which individual funds may levy contributions from their members (*Hochstsatz*). The tax rate is expressed as a percentage of the wage base. Each sickness fund sets its own rate (*Beitragssatz*), and there is great variation in the rates charged by the different sickness funds. In 1978, the rates varied between 7 percent and 14.2 percent—a twofold difference.[29] Factory sickness funds exhibit the greatest range of rates of all fund types, which is not surprising since they tend to be smaller than the other types, and since they are likely to concentrate members who share the same occupation-specific risks.

Because the rates charged depend partly on the expenditures that must be covered by each fund (and thus on the health of a fund's members) and partly on the income of fund members (i.e., the total taxable wage base available for taxation), it is inevitable that an insurance system based on separate groups will have to use different tax rates. From some points of view, differential tax rates are indicative of distributive inequity.[30] However, differential tax rates for insurance premiums are "inequitable" only against a standard of universal insurance, in which the risks are pooled across the entire nation.

The dynamics of health insurance financing have been patently regressive. Until 1971, the legislature increased the taxable wage base infrequently. Between 1904 and 1971, it was raised only ten times (see table 5.7). The inflexibility of the wage base meant that

Table 5.7 Changes in Minimum Income Level for Exemption from Compulsory Insurance

Year	Exemption Level (RM/DM)
1904	2,000
1914	2,500
1925	2,700
1927	3,600
1949	4,500
1952	6,000
1957	7,920
1965	10,800
1969	11,880
1970	14,400
1971*	17,100
1977	30,600

Note: * As of 1971, the exemption level is raised automatically each year. Source: Bundesministerium für Arbeit und Sozialordnung, *Übersicht über die Soziale Sicherung*, 1977, p. 185.

sickness funds had to increase their tax rate in order to meet increased expenditures. The government quietly allowed the nominal ceiling on the tax rate to be exceeded. During the 1960s, the maximum rate was 11 percent. With the transfer of liability for wage continuation payments from sickness funds to employers in 1970, the maximum tax rate was reduced to 8 percent. But by 1973, the average rate charged by sickness funds was up to 9 percent.[31] By avoiding increases in the taxable wage base, the legislature effectively protected the incomes of middle and high income earners. As average wages rose and the taxable wage base remained fixed, more income of people in the middle and high ranges would become exempt from the social insurance tax. Meanwhile, people earning below the wage base amount were required to pay ever increasing proportions of their income in social security taxes.

Given the incentives of elected politicians, it is not surprising that the legislature adopted this strategy. Increasing revenue by holding down the wage base and allowing the tax rate to rise concentrates the costs on people at the low end of the income distribution, who are also relatively uninfluential politically. On the other hand, since any increase in this level draws more people out of private insurance and increases employer contributions to premiums, there is also pressure against increasing the level. As of 1971, the wage base/minimum earnings level was pegged to national wage levels, and is now automatically increased every year, so the political tension for the legislature is gone.

The Double-Edged Sword of Lower Costs

One indicator of the effectiveness of funds is the cost of health care to their members compared with the cost to privately insured or self-paying patients. In fact, the sickness funds do pay lower prices for almost all medical services. Office-based physicians are paid according to separate fee schedules for the different types of funds, and it has been estimated that the fees paid by private patients are on average double those paid by the RVO funds for their members.[32] Fund patients also pay less for drugs and for hospital services than private patients. The funds are given quantity discounts by the pharmacies; one study estimated the average size of the discount to be about seven percent.[33] As of 1976, the discount is 5 percent. Finally, the daily rate that hospitals were allowed to charge sickness funds was lower than the rate for private patients, but since 1972, rates have been the same.

The paradox of procurement at lower costs is that the funds are often accused of providing "second class medicine." In a sense, the funds are in a no-win situation: if they do not secure services for their members at prices lower than the private market prices, they have no reason for existence as a social institution. Patients might as well insure through commercial insurance companies. On the other hand, if they do procure services at lower prices, many people think that they are providing a lower standard of care.

There is very little empirical evidence about actual quality differences in the services received by privately and publicly insured patients. A national study commission in 1966 claimed that office physicians practice different styles of medicine for fund and private patients and that the average duration of a physician visit for a private patient is longer than for a fund patient.[34] It is well known that many office physicians provide certain amenities for their private patients, such as scheduled appointment times instead of the usual open office hours, shorter waiting times for appointments, and separate waiting rooms.[35] Within the hospital, private insurance will cover single rooms, while public insurance covers only semiprivate and ward accommodations. Whether these differences in "styles" are really just differences in amenities or actual differences in quality is hard to resolve. In any case, much of the efficacy of medical care derives from the psychological reassurance patients receive, and if amenities contribute to that reassurance, they might well be considered an aspect of the "quality of care."

This point is well illustrated by answers to a survey in 1973. The most common complaint about the health care system was waiting time in physicians' offices. When asked to estimate how long they usually have to wait to see their physician, respondents' answers varied with the type of insurance they held: the average self-reported waiting time was 78 minutes for members of local sickness funds, 64 minutes for members of substitute funds, and 43 minutes for private patients. When asked how long the physician usually spends with them, however, respondents' answers were generally uniform (about 19 minutes), with no variation by type of insurance. Yet 54 percent of the respondents believed that "in general, physicians give more effort for private patients than for sickness fund patients."[36]

Thus, there is a widespread popular belief that a dual standard of care exists, and this belief alone is a strong force with which policymakers must reckon.[37] Private insurance companies and substitute funds are able to play on the popular conception that higher priced services are of higher quality. Their advertisements subtly utilize the notion that they provide "better" care. When physicians tell a patient that his fund will not pay for a certain medicine, the impression of a dual standard is reinforced. The public insurance system thus has a difficult mandate—to provide people with services of the same scope and quality as privately insured persons receive, but at a lower total cost. This is certainly a fundamental dilemma of any national health insurance program whenever a legitimate private market for health services is allowed to coexist with it.

Limits on Collective Power: Reimbursement Methods | Chapter Six

Methods of physician reimbursement can potentially serve as a means of control over the quantity and types of services provided. Since 1932, when the system of direct negotiations between sickness funds and AIDs was consolidated, the system of physician reimbursement has been a two-stage process. In the first stage, the sickness funds pay the AIDs an aggregate pool in exchange for all the services provided to fund members. In the second stage, the AIDs distribute the pool to their individual physician members. The distribution of the pool is based on a fee schedule and the individual service claims submitted by the physicians. Decisions for each of the two stages—setting the size of the total pool and determining the prices for individual fees—have traditionally been made through some kind of bargaining process between the sickness funds and the AIDs. These collective negotiations are intended to put some constraints on the discretionary power of physicians to determine the total volume and mix of medical services.

Determination of the Pool

Before 1932, the sickness funds' method of payment to physicians was only loosely regulated.[1] The Berlin Treaty of 1913 explicitly left the payment method to the determination of individual contracts between physicians and funds. During the 1920s, the emergency orders reiterated the principle that relations between funds and physicians were a matter for private contracts, and allowed the funds to choose from any of several payment methods.

The regulations of 1931 and 1932, which created the system of AIDs and collective contracts, also established a single method of payment. Sickness funds were to pay the AIDs an aggregate reimbursement or pool (*Gesamtvergütung*), and the AIDs were to be responsible for distributing the pool to their members. The only permissible method for establishing the pool was a prospectively set capitation (or per person) fee. Because the funds were experiencing serious financial difficulties during this period, the regulations (issued by the Ministry of Labory) also stated that the size of the capitation fee had to take into account "special conditions" and the "general economic circumstances" of the sickness fund. The size of the capitation fee was specifically allowed to vary with changes in a sickness fund's taxable wage base.[2]

In a major reform of 1955 (the Kassenarztrecht), the RVO was modified to allow sickness funds to choose any of several methods of calculating the pool, including fee-for-service, a fee per visit (*Fallpauschale*), the older capitation method, and mixed forms. In addition, the new rules specified that even under a capitation method, the sickness funds had to take into account changes in the volume of physicians' services. The provision for a fee-for-service method of setting the pool was not part of the original bill submitted to the legislature and was added only during conference in the Bundestag. Fee-for-service was simply mentioned as a possibility, but the method was not worked out in any detail, since everyone thought that capitation would remain the predominant method of payment.[3]

For several years, the funds continued to negotiate their pools on a capitation basis. Gradually, a few funds switched to the fee-for-service method. The first fund to switch did not do so until 1958, and by 1965 only a small group of funds had switched. Then, between 1965 and 1968, virtually all of the RVO funds switched to the fee-for-service method of determining the pool.

Under this new method, physicians' fees are set in advance (by the fee schedule), but the size of the pool can be determined only at the end of a payment period, by multiplying the actual volume of services by their respective prices.[4] The size of the pool is still supposed to take into account "the financial condition of the fund," but the law provides no firm criteria for exactly how this is to be done, or even how a fund's financial condition is to be measured. And since a fund can always enhance its financial position by raising its tax rate, pegging the size of the pool to a fund's financial strength hardly gives the funds any leverage over physicians in controlling expenditures.[5]

The question of whether the funds should use a capitation or a fee-for-service method of setting the pool was a major debate in social insurance policy in the 1960s.[6] Physicians insisted that only a fee-for-service system was equitable, because any other system did not pay them according to the work they actually performed. Sickness fund administrators pointed out that the current capitation system, modified as it was by the volume of services, was really an "indirect fee-for-service method" and that through the distribution of the pool, physicians' actual fees were indeed commensurate with the value of services rendered. Physicians argued that any prospective method of setting the pool would penalize them for increases in morbidity and consequent increases in services. The sickness funds responded that physicians actually control the volume of services to a large degree, and they *should* be at risk for those services that are not strictly medically necessary. As one administrator said: "The sickness funds ask themselves how things will look under a fee-for-service system, whereby, in their view, expansion of the scope of medical services has no limits. Such fears are certainly not unfounded."[7]

There was considerable popular support for a switch to the fee-for-service method for setting the pool. The substitute funds had switched to that method, and the popular press played upon the idea that the RVO funds, because they used a different method, must be providing "welfare medicine." Fritz Kastner, the director of the Federal Association of Local Sickness Funds at the time, thought that the popular support for fee-for-service derived from a widespread misunderstanding of the existing system.[8] He thought that the public was particularly susceptible to physicians' claims that they were not being paid equitably, because it did not understand that physician payment occurred in two stages and that the individual physician's payment was determined by a fee-for-service method. Meanwhile, some newspapers claimed that the doctor/patient relationship was more "trusting" in regions where the sickness funds had switched to fee-for-service.[9] The whole issue of determination of the pool became in the public debate one of two-class medicine. Cost control was again a double-edged sword.

The transition to the fee-for-service method of setting the size of the pool was clearly a tremendous boon to physicians, yet the reasons for the switch and the conflicts that must have ensued have remained a mystery, even in German social science literature. When the issue is discussed at all, the change is usually rationalized as a means of providing the sickness funds with more leverage over physicians. With the detailed records on individual procedures required by the fee-for-service system, the funds can monitor physicians' behavior more closely. Since they receive claims forms that itemize all procedures, they can assess the appropriateness of individual services and find out from patients whether the services claimed were actually provided.[10] But, as Kastner wrote in 1965, sickness funds already had statutory authority to monitor physicians' services, and there was no reason why they could not have collected the same data under the capitation method.[11]

In 1965, when only about sixty funds had switched to fee-for-service, Kastner proposed that these funds be considered a natural experiment, and that other funds wait several years to evaluate the results before rushing to make the switch themselves.[12] But fee-for-service became the "prestigious method," as it was the one used by the substitute funds, so that the individual RVO funds were increasingly pressured to switch, even though the fund association leaders knew that the switch would have disastrous consequences for sickness fund cost control efforts. In the next three years there was something of a bandwagon, and by 1968 virtually all the funds had changed to the fee-for-service method.

By 1970, the two-stage method of payment that had originally served to place a ceiling on expenditures for physicians' services had become simply a complex way of reimbursing physicians on a fee-for-service basis, while preserving the role of AIDs as fiscal intermediaries. Under the old system, the size of the pool was relatively fixed, and the physicians were thus involved in a zero-sum game with each other. Since they were competing for the same limited pot of money, they all had an incentive to monitor each other's claims. Under the fee-for-service method of setting the pool, each physician could increase his claims infinitely without reducing the income of his fellow physicians.

Besides eliminating the constraint on total expenditures for physicians' services, the new method of setting the pool had an additional advantage for physicians. Under the old capitation-based method, the main way for physicians as a group to obtain a higher income from the funds (i.e., a larger pool) was to have the minimum income for exemption raised, so that more people would be insured in the public system and capitation payments would be increased. But such an increase could be obtained only at the expense of the private sector—the more people in the public insurance system, the fewer in the private insurance system, and thus the lower the income physicians could generate through their private, fee-for-service practice. Under the new fee-for-service method of setting the pool, physicians can increase their income from the sickness funds by bargaining for higher fees, by providing more services per patient, or by providing a more expensive mix of services, all without trading off any income from their privately insured patients.

Determination of Fees

Once the pool has been paid by a sickness fund to an AID, the AID must distribute the money among its individual members. The distribution is done on a fee-for-service basis. Physicians submit a claim for every patient, stating the fund membership of the patient and listing the services provided. The fees used to determine actual physician reimbursement levels are derived from fee schedules negotiated by the sickness funds and the AIDs.

The fee schedules actually comprise two separate elements. First, a series of relative value scales (*Verteilungsmaßstäbe*) establish the relative values of the several hundred procedures performed by office-based physicians. Each medical procedure is assigned a point value. The purpose of the schedules is to establish a ranking of medical procedures according to their labor, capital, and time costs as well as technical difficulty. These scales are the fee schedules proper.

Second, the sickness funds and AIDs negotiate conversion factors (*Honorarsätze*) annually. The conversion factors determine the monetary value of points in the fee schedules, and are generally applied across-the-board to all procedures in the fee schedules. For example, a point is currently worth about 10 Pfennig. Different conversion factors are negotiated for each type of sickness fund and each region.

Relative value scales may be created either by Parliament or by contract between the sickness funds and the AIDs. Contractual schedules are much more flexible instruments. They can be changed as often as necessary, whereas a statutory schedule can be changed only through a lengthy legislative process. Also, contractual schedules allow for periodic revaluation of individual procedures, but Parliament cannot possibly provide continual updating of relative values.

There are several different relative value scales governing the relationships between the different types of funds and the AIDs. Until 1965, the RVO funds paid according to the old "Preugo," a fee schedule established by the Reichstag in 1896. The substitute funds used the "E-ADGO," a contractual schedule established in 1929.[13] In the late 1950s, as part of a general reform effort in health insurance, the federal government attempted to introduce a fee schedule with a relative value scale more in accord with the realities of modern medicine. For several years, the labor and health ministries struggled with each other over control of the new fee schedule. The conflict resulted in a stalemate, and the new statutory schedule that was finally passed in 1965 was a compromise: it was neither a totally new revaluation of procedures, nor a linear increase in the Preugo, but rather simply an adoption of a previously existing schedule used by the substitute funds.[14] This new statutory schedule, the Gebührenordnung-Ärzte or GOÄ, was meant to be a transitional schedule to update the old Preugo until a more thorough restructuring could be agreed upon. But since 1965, there has been no new statutory schedule, and the sickness funds have concluded several contractual schedules based on the GOÄ. The two most important such schedules are the Bewertungsmaßstab-Ärzte, or BMÄ, which is negotiated between the federal associations of each type of RVO fund and the Federal Association of Insurance Doctors (KBV) to govern payment for services rendered to RVO fund members; and the Allgemeine Deutsche Gebührenordnung-Ersatzkassen or E-ADGO, negotiated between the substitute funds and the Federal Association of Insurance Doctors to govern payments for services rendered to substitute fund members. Negotiating committees for the respective parties to these contracts meet quite frequently (at least several times a year) to discuss revaluation of particular procedures.

In addition to the negotiations over the relative value scales, there are continuing and even more complex negotiations over the conversion factors. These negotiations are in general very decentralized. Although the sickness funds are legally permitted to bargain individually with the AIDs, the RVO funds mostly bargain at the *Land* level. In general, each type of fund (i.e., local, factory, guild, agricultural) conducts its own negotiations.[15] Thus, at any time, the *Land*-level AID may be conducting negotiations with the *Land* association of each type of RVO fund. In 1971, the Federal Association of RVO Funds began negotiating national guidelines (the *Bundesmantelvertrag*) for the regional contracts, but the primary negotiations still remain at the *Land* level. And to make matters more complicated, in some areas the RVO funds and AIDs continue to negotiate slight increases in the conversion factors for regions smaller than the *Länder*.

Outside of the RVO funds, the negotiations over conversion factors are generally held on the national level. The federal associations of substitute funds for white-collar and blue-collar workers bargain together with the· Federal Association of Insurance Doctors. In addition, several separate insurance programs for government employees also negotiate on the natural level. Thus, the Federal Association of Insurance Doctors contracts with the Ministry of Defense (for coverage of armed services personnel), the Ministry of Labor (for civil servants), and the Ministry of the Interior (for the border patrol).

For the purposes of administering the payment of physicians, the AIDs operate multiple accounting branches within each *Land*.

Each physician submits his claims to the appropriate regional accounting unit. The claims forms are the vouchers that have been received from patients, and each voucher contains space for the physician to record dates, diagnoses, and procedures. For all practical purposes, the AIDs use the same relative value scale to determine the distribution of the pool as the physicians use to submit their claims for payment. But several other factors are used to determine the ultimate individual reimbursements, and certain costs other than physicians' fees must be paid out of the total pool received from the AID.

From the total pool, the AID makes certain deductions to cover its operating costs and special programs. The most important special programs are a disability and survivors' insurance program for physicians, for which deductions are taken automatically from the pool; special subsidies to physicians who establish a practice in underdoctored areas; special subsidies to provide elderly physicians with a guaranteed minimum income; and payments to physicians for providing coverage during holidays, Sundays, and nights.[16] Some operating costs may also be deducted from the total pool, but most administrative expenses are covered by charging each physician a flat percentage (usually 2–3 percent) of his total reimbursement each quarter.[17] When all these deductions have been made, the remaining sum is the total divisible pool.

Under the old capitation-based system of setting the pool in advance, the value of the pool was usually less than the total value of physicians' claims according to the fee schedule and conversion factors (see table 6.1). In this case, all physicians' payments were reduced in proportion to the ratio of the pool value to total claims value. For example, if the ratio of the pool to total claims was .80, then each fee-for-service claim would be honored using only 80 percent of the prevailing conversion factor value. This system of "discounting" physicians' claims (*Quotierung*) gradually disappeared as more and more funds agreed to calculate the pool directly from the fee-for-service claims.

The Impact of Reimbursement Methods on Priorities in Service Delivery

If the countervailing power strategy were truly effective, one would expect the sickness funds to be able to influence the mix of services provided by manipulating the relative value scales. There is general agreement among officials in the health sector that the fee schedules overvalue technical procedures relative to personal procedures. Much of what physicians do involves spending time talking with patients, questioning, advising, explaining, instructing, and reassuring. But the fee schedules list primarily technical procedures (injections, fracture reduction, dressing wounds, and so on), and the only way a physician can bill for time he spends talking with a patient is to use either the "consultation" or "thorough examination" items, which have very low relative values of DM 3.00 and 6.70 respectively. In the 1973 BMÄ, containing several hundred items, there were only twelve that were valued lower.[18] By comparison, numerous technical procedures under the category "physical medicine" reimburse at the same rate or higher. Physical medicine procedures, such as whirlpool or hydroelectric baths, are performed primarily by technical assistants and involve little if any of a physician's time. Diagnostic and therapeutic radiology, which again involve primarily technician time, is another category that is extremely highly reimbursed.

The relative values for radiology and physical medicine reflect, of course, the substantial capital investment required in these particular fields. But the issue for reformers in West Germany is whether the fee schedule creates incentives for overcapitalization of office-based practices. The problem of creating a schedule that properly reflects the importance of personal interaction between

Table 6.1 Ratio of Payments by Sickness Funds (AID pool) to Total Physician Claims

Year	Ratio
1958	.792
1959	.847
1960	.889
1961	.913
1962	.951
1963	.973
1964	1.039
1965	.851
1966	.965
1967	.988
1968	1.002
1969	1.032
1970	1.095

Source: *Statistisches Jahrbuch der Kassenärztlichen Bundesvereinigung 1971* (Köln, 1971), tables 63 and 65. Data are for RVO funds only.

doctor and patient but also enables physicians to purchase and maintain the necessary capital equipment is considered extremely important by officials of all the organizations concerned with health insurance, but there is as yet no hard data on the actual costs of office-based practice and the incentives created by the schedules.

Because the fee schedules create different rewards for different patterns of capitalization of medical practice, they might be expected to engender strong interests among subgroups of the medical profession. A group that has made a heavy investment in one kind of technology (and one kind of training) will naturally have an intense interest in the portion of the fee schedule that applies to its specialty or area of practice. Moreover, the process by which the fee schedules are established—i.e., the AIDs, representing all insurance doctors, bargain with the sickness funds—is more political than technical, thus giving much weight to the strength and intensity of physician preferences and relatively little weight to objective analyses of the time and money costs of the individual procedures. The process may also have a bandwagon effect. Once a particular technology becomes relatively profitable within the structure of the fee schedule, physicians will have a strong economic incentive to invest in it further, as will physicians as they set up new practices. As the financial investment in the technology grows, so will the political sentiment against altering the relative values of the fee schedule.[19]

Most analysts of the West German health system agree that a process of this nature is responsible for the relatively heavy investment in and use of therapeutic radiation machines by office-based physicians. Almost half of all specialists other than radiologists and nearly a fifth of all general practitioners have radiation equipment in their offices.[20] In 1975, the mean value of capital equipment and office space per practice was about DM 34,000, of which about DM 9,000 (or more than 25%) was for X-ray equipment. And between 1971 and 1975, the value of X-ray equipment per practice jumped 87 percent.[21]

In addition, there is real concern among government and fund officials that the incentives created by the fee schedules to purchase capital equipment then lead physicians to overutilize the equipment. An intensive government study of radiology found some alarming results. While internists without radiation equipment recommend a referral to a radiologist in only two percent of their cases, internists with radiation equipment deem X-rays necessary in fifteen percent of their cases. Similarly, pediatricians without the equipment refer only five percent of their patients for X-rays, but those with equipment find X-rays necessary for twenty-five percent of their patients. Gynecologists with mammography equipment X-ray fully fifty percent of their patients, despite expert opinion that mammography is warranted in only about ten to twenty percent of adult women. The higher figures for physicians with radiology equipment in part reflect the fact that they receive referrals from the physicians without equipment. But the large discrepancies have led to questions about the extent of unnecessary radiation by office-based physicians.[22]

For several years, the sickness fund administrators and many officials in the Ministry of Labor have promoted an upward revaluation of procedures that require relatively more physician time and a corresponding devaluation of procedures that physicians commonly delegate to assistants and that involve the use of machines more than physician time. The substitute funds took the lead in restructuring their relative value scales, with a major revaluation of consultations, visits, and examinations between 1970 and 1972 (see table 6.2).[23] The RVO funds followed suit, and in the federal guidelines (*Bundesmantelvertrag*) of 1975, laboratory procedures were devalued by twenty-five percent and personal procedures were revalued upward by about forty-five percent.

Evidence about the change in mix of services provided by physicians suggests that the relative value scales will have to be changed drastically to reverse or alter the trend toward more and

Table 6.2 Restructuring of Relative Values in E-ADGO

Procedure	Relative Value 1963	Index of Procedure Values (1963=100)			
		1967	1970	1971	1972
Consultation	3	125	125	138.30	166.67
Home visit- daytime	6	125	187.5	206.67	206.67
Thorough examination	5	125	167.0	184.00	184.00
Psychotherapy	30	125	125	200.00	200.00
All Surgical procedures[a]		125	125	137.50	171.85
All Laboratory Procedures[a]		125	125	137.50	137.50

Note: [a] Composite index.
Source: Gesellschaft für Sozialen Fortschritt, *Der Wandel der Stellung des Arztes im Einkommensgefüge* (Bonn, 1974), p. 66.

more diagnostic, laboratory, and radiology procedures (see table 6.3). Diagnostic tests now account for twenty-five percent of the expenditures of sickness funds, and X-rays account for fully twelve percent.

The fee schedules, because they are created by a process of negotiation between physicians' associations and sickness funds, and because they are the basis for all reimbursement of physicians, are a clear means by which the collective action of physicians creates a reward structure that can influence the diagnostic and therapeutic decisions of individual physicians in individual cases. Here it is not even necessary to assume that these decisions are at all motivated or determined by economic considerations. The reward structure of the fee schedule may have a profound influence on the investment decisions of physicians—how they choose to equip their offices—and thus on the range of options from which they choose diagnostic and therapeutic procedures at the level of the individual case.

The creation of fee schedules through negotiations between physicians' organizations and sickness funds is potentially a way that large consumer membership organizations could influence the mix of medical services provided. The persistence of a relatively high valuation of technical procedures that are relatively

Table 6.3 Changes in Service Mix of Office-Based Physicians

	1965		1974	
Service	Average Claim per Case (DM)	Percent of Total Claim per Case	Average Claim per Case (DM)	Percent of Total Claim per Case
Consultations	7.70	31.2%	7.31	20.0%
Visits	2.06	8.3	1.55	4.2
Minor medical procedures	7.53	30.5	10.42	28.5
Diagnostic tests/ procedures	2.56	10.4	9.13	25.0
Medical supplies	1.33	5.4	1.69	4.6
X-rays	2.45	9.9	4.65	12.7
Total claim	24.68	100.0	36.59	100.0

Note: "Case" refers to a voucher, and therefore includes all services for a patient in a three-month period. A case may include more than one visit or more than one medical problem.
Source: Theo Siebeck, *Zur Kostenentwicklung in der Krankenversicherung* (Bonn: Verlag der Ortskrankenkassen, 1976), p. 87.

cheap to produce leads one to be quite pessimistic about the ability of even large patient organizations to alter the reward structure of medical care. On the other hand, the changes that have been introduced in some fee schedules indicate the possibilities for change through the countervailing power strategy.

Chapter Seven | Limits on Discretionary Power: Economic Monitoring

Under national health insurance and other kinds of third-party payment programs, the discretionary decisions of physicians about their patients' medical needs become spending decisions of the government or other payors. In medical care programs, where individual needs can be determined only by technical experts, the third-party payors are dependent on physicians to make judgments about what services should be purchased for the members. The payors, whether they are insurance companies (and ultimately their policyholders) or government agencies (and ultimately the taxpayers) therefore have little control over their own budgets. If they wish to place any kind of constraints on individual physicians' ability to order unlimited medical care, they have two possible mechanisms. One is simply to limit the total amount of money available for medical services. As we saw in chapter 6, the German sickness funds abandoned the element of fixed budgeting through a capitation-based, prospectively negotiated pool. In the absence of a total budget constraint, third-party payors must establish standards of benefit coverage and somehow review all service claims to determine whether the services are justified according to the standards. The West German national health insurance program uses a system called "economic monitoring" (*Wirtschaftlichkeitsprüfung*) to set standards and review services.

The debate over the scope of "unnecessary services" that has taken place in the United States only during the past ten years began far earlier in Germany. Already in 1927, the physician Erwin Liek estimated that two-thirds of the services performed by physicians were unnecessary.[1]

The motivation for some kind of utilization review of medical services has changed over time, as the payment mechanism has changed, and as the financial strength of the sickness funds has changed. Before the institution of collective negotiations for a fixed pool, the sickness funds had some control over expenditures for physicians' services in that most contracts with physicians set a fixed salary. But salaries gave the funds no leverage over the cost of drugs and appliances prescribed by their physicians. In 1923, a period of rapid inflation and financial difficulty for the sickness funds, an emergency order obligated insurance doctors to refrain from unnecessary treatment and to limit prescriptions to those absolutely necessary. Repeated violations of this injunction could lead to a suspension of the permit for insurance practice. Another emergency order in 1931 eventually allowed the sickness funds to hold physicians liable for the costs of excess or unnecessary services.[2]

Beginning in 1932, when the system of collective negotiations over a capitation-based pool was established, the incentives for utilization review shifted. Since each AID was furnished with a fixed pool of money to distribute, and since individual physicians could make potentially unlimited claims on the pool, the AIDs and their members began to use utilization review as a method for controlling the distribution of the pool. Since 1968, when most of the sickness funds had switched to a fee-for-service method of calculating the pool, the incentives for control have switched back to the funds. Because the funds cannot put a ceiling on expenditures, they need to be able to control their own expenditures. Controlling increases in fees is not enough if physicians can manipulate the volume of services.

The Legal Basis for Economic Monitoring

Economic monitoring occurs during the second stage of social insurance payment, the distribution of the quarterly pool received by the AIDs to their individual members. Distribution of the pool is entirely the prerogative of the AIDs, but the system of distribution must follow certain standards set forth in the RVO (section 368f). The distribution must be based on the nature and quantity of services provided by each physician. Since 1958 the AIDs have been expressly prohibited from paying a flat rate per voucher. During World War II, a reimbursement system based on a fee per voucher was used, and many people believe the voucher system is still in effect. Some patients allegedly offer to give physicians extra vouchers, thinking that the physician will be paid more and that they will receive better care.[3] The method of distribution must also assure that physicians will not "overextend" themselves in their practice. This provision was first introduced in 1931, at the same time as the ratio of sickness fund doctors to insured persons was lowered to 1:600. The funds have always perceived a close connection between the number of doctors in a community and the number of services provided.

The exact meaning of "overextension of practice" (*übermässige Ausdehnung der Praxis*) is not defined in the law, but has evolved more through the practice of the AIDs and litigation in the courts. In practice, overextension seems to mean performing too many services in the aggregate. Until recently, the AIDs used schedules of declining marginal fees (*Ertragstaffeln*), such that the price per service earned by a physician declined as the number of services went up. An example of such a schedule might be:

for 1 to 600 cases   maximum of DM x per case
for 601 to 800 cases   maximum of DM x-0.50 per case
for 801 to 100 cases   maximum of DM x-1 per case.[4]

Physicians have been intensely opposed to the use of aggregate schedules and have constantly challenged their legality. A decision of the social court in Stuttgart in 1959 found several justifications for the schedules: they protect the funds against "fund-hogs" who would overdoctor in order to maximize their own income; they protect the patient against low-quality and ineffective care, insofar as overextension means that a physician does not devote enough time and care to medical decisions, and that he is overworked and therefore not mentally alert.[5] The Berlin Social Court in 1961 also thought the schedules were justified because they make physicians consider the true value of services more carefully.[6] Most, but not all, state-level social courts affirmed the legality of the categorical schedules; the Federal Social Court in 1965 decided that the schedules were permissible as long as they could be reasonably shown to bear on community welfare.

In 1972, the issue was appealed to the Supreme Constitutional Court, which overturned the earlier decisions on the grounds of insufficient evidence to prove the alleged benefits of the schedules. Many physicians argue that the schedules are unreasonable because they do not differentiate between different specialties or between different kinds of services which take varying amounts of time. Schedules that make such differentiations are currently in use and have been upheld by various district social courts.[7]

Undoubtedly the conflict over controls on overextension of practice is fundamentally a conflict between physicians who perform primarily time-consuming, labor-intensive personal procedures (most primary care phsyicians, such as general practitioners, pediatricians, internists, obstetricians, and gynecologists) and physicians in specialties that use a high proportion of technical and mechanical procedures. Whereas the technical specialties seem to be better able to control the structure of the fee schedules, the procedures for review of overextension may be the weapon of the primary care physicians. In any case, the use and type of overextension controls apparently varies widely among the many regional AIDs, and the impact of these controls on social expenditures for health services or on physicians' incomes is difficult to assess.

Economic monitoring differs theoretically from the overextension controls in that it seeks to review the quality of services in individual cases. By contrast, the overextension controls merely assume a relationship between quantity and quality of services and impose controls strictly on the basis of quantity. The legal basis for economic monitoring of doctors' behavior is found in two sections of the Imperial Insurance Code. In the section on entitlements of insured persons during illness, the law states: "Medical care must be sufficient and appropriate; it must not, however, exceed the limits of what is necessary" (section 182, part 2). This provision derives from the initial conception of national health insurance as providing minimal necessary care for industrial workers. In the section of the RVO dealing with the rights of physicians and their relationships to funds and patients, the patients' rights are defined more liberally:

> The insured person is entitled to care that is appropriate and sufficient for a cure or relief according to the standards of medical practice. Services which are not necessary or economical for the accomplishment of a successful cure may not be claimed by the insured; the insurance doctor or participating doctor must not perform or order such services; the fund may not approve them ex post facto. [section 368c]

Physicians have constantly challenged economic monitoring in the courts. In 1962, the Association of Office-Based Physicians (NÄV) brought a case to the Supreme Constitutional Court, in which the association claimed that the standards articulated in the RVO were "elastic, and therefore unable to guarantee a protection of rights." The court rejected the claim, saying that physicians have an obligation to practice economically even in their private practices.[8] In another case in the same year, the Federal Social Court rejected an argument that the standards in the two parts of the RVO were inconsistent; it held that the principle of "economy" as a standard for economic monitoring subsumed the principles of "sufficient, appropriate, and not exceeding that which is necessary."[9]

In 1965, the Federal Social Court extended the entitlement of insured persons even further. It held that the concept of sufficient care has two sides. On the one hand, the physician can be denied payment for unnecessary or uneconomical services. On the other hand, the physician is obligated "to provide the insured person with care that is appropriate and sufficient, i.e., thorough and careful [*gründlich und sorgfältig*]."[10] This decision changed the character of the entitlement from a minimal definition, designed to exclude many services, to a maximal definition, designed to include most services. The legal standard of "economical care," against which physicians' services are reviewed, has thus become synonymous with the customary standard of care in the medical community.

Responsibility for conducting economic monitoring used to rest almost entirely with the AIDs, since the review of services was conducted as part of the distribution of the pool:

> In order to control the economy [*Wirtschaftlichkeit*] of medical care by insurance doctors, the associations of insurance doctors will form, according to the more precise terms of their own bylaws, monitoring and grievance committees, insofar as the pool is not calculated on a fee-for-service basis. [RVO section 368n(4)]

The sickness funds were entitled to send representatives to the AID review committees, but only as consultants, not as voting members. With the transition to a fee-for-service method of setting the pool, the funds had a more pressing interest in conducting economic monitoring, because the claims of individual physicians now directly affected the size of the pool. The RVO was revised to give sickness funds slightly more weight in economic monitoring:

> If the pool is calculated on a fee-for-service basis, the composition of the committees and their methods for reviewing physicians' services shall be determined by agreement between the parties to the contract [i.e., funds and AIDs]. [section 368n(5)]

In practice, there has been a great variety in the composition of monitor committees, ranging from the sickness funds' having only one member with voting rights, to parity and a rotating chairmanship. Generally, the AIDs retained a majority on the monitor committees until 1977.

The Mechanics of Economic Monitoring

The essence of the peer review system is the computation of various average claims (in DM) for all physicians and comparison of individual physician's average claims with group averages.[11] The initial comparisons are used to screen out cases where there is a large deviation for closer scrutiny. These cases are then examined to establish whether there is a valid reason for the deviation. If none can be found, an adjustment (or cutback) will be made in the physician's reimbursement.

The averages are constructed for about ten categories of services and procedures:

—Consultations

—Visits (house calls)

—General services (written reports, letters to other physicians or hospitals, sick leave certificates)

—Special services (all diagnostic and therapeutic services, except physician therapy, radiology, and laboratory tests; special services may be further subdivided into "small" and "large" categories, using some fixed monetary value as a dividing line.)

—Physical therapy (massages, whirlpools, baths, exercises)

—Radiology (sometimes further divided into diagnostic and therapeutic radiology)

—Laboratory tests

—Travel allowances (special fees for mileage)

—In-hospital services (for office-based physicians with staff privileges)

Each doctor's cases are also separated according to the sickness fund of the patient. For example, separate average per patient claims are developed for all patients in the agricultural fund, in the factory funds, in the guild funds, and so on. This is because the different funds pay slightly different benefits. If, for example, one fund in the region paid for flu vaccinations and a doctor had a high number of patients from that fund, his average cost per patient in the category of special services would be elevated by the many flu vaccinations.

Finally, physicians are separated by specialty, and sometimes further divided into more homogeneous comparison groups. Each doctor is compared only with doctors of the same specialty in the same region, and general practitioners are compared only with each other. In the case of very rare specialties, or of a doctor with relatively rare equipment in his office, he is compared with averages developed for the entire *Land*.

Physicians' challenges of the economic monitoring system have generally been centered on claims that the AIDs did not use the appropriate comparison group for an individual physician, and consequently there has been a great deal of decisionmaking by the social courts on the mechanics of constructing comparison groups. In general, the courts have sustained the position of the AIDs that group comparisons are the only practical method of conducting economic monitoring, and that review of individual physicians' claims without reference to group averages would be unfeasible. The courts have said that the reference group must be "comparable" and that simply separating physicians by specialty may not always be refined enough. The AIDs must take into account the characteristics of a physician's practice, which include diagnostic and therapeutic equipment, and the proportion of referrals from other physicians offering similar services in the community.[12]

An average claim per case (based on fee schedule values) is calculated for each category of specialist and each category of medical services.[13] The AID then prepares an overview (*Gesamtübersicht*) of each doctor's claim for the quarter, including the physician's *total claim* and *average claim per case* for each category of medical service; the *average claim per case* for the specialty as a whole, and for a smaller reference group when appropriate, for each category of service; the *average number of cases* for the physician and for relevant reference groups; the *difference* between the average claim per case of the individual doctor and the group averages (specialty and/or reference group) for each category of service. Each of these values is calculated separately for patients with different insurance statuses, such as pensioners, contributing members and dependents, and members of RVO funds and substitute funds.

The different AIDs use slightly different measures of the *difference* between a physician's claims and group average claims. The majority express the difference as a simple percentage, so that a physician would be selected for further scrutiny if his claims were greater than 140 percent, 160 percent, or 200 percent of the average claims value. (The exact criterion is set by each AID.) Other AIDs use other measures, such as the mean deviation, the mean squared deviation, or the standard deviation. Whatever the exact criterion, however, the important feature is that all economic monitoring uses the *average claim* as a basic standard.

Certain additional information is compiled for each doctor. A service chart (*Leistungsnachweis*) is prepared, showing, for every case (each of which is assigned a case number), the total fees claimed for each of the categories of service, as well as the total fees claimed for that case. In addition, a checklist (*Prüfkarte*) is submitted by each doctor. This describes the important features of his practice that may have a bearing on his costs and claims. The card describes the location of the practice, whether the doctor also has hospital privileges, any special office apparatus (such as ray lamps, whirlpools, exercise machines, inhalation therapy equipment, electrocardiographs, and so on), laboratory facilities, X-ray equipment, and any other special features of the practice.

All of this information is then handed over to a monitor doctor (*Prüfarzt*). Monitor doctors are practicing insurance doctors who are paid by the AID to review cases. The monitor checks through the doctors one at a time. He first looks at the overview to determine whether the doctor has exceeded the group average by more than the set tolerance limit in any of the service categories. If he finds an excess, he then looks for more information to determine whether there are mitigating circumstances, such as a large number of pensioners, a large number of patients in a particular fund, coverage of another doctor's practice during vacation or illness, or an epidemic in the region. The doctor might have some special equipment uncommon in the region which accounts for a high claim in a particular category. Finally, if the monitor doctor cannot find a general circumstance to justify the excessive claim, he can look at the service chart to see if the excesses are due to (or at least limited to) a few individual cases. By looking up the claims forms for those few cases, he can then judge whether the procedures and treatments were "sufficient, appropriate, economical, and necessary," given the diagnosis listed by the physician.

The monitor doctor makes allowances for all the mitigating circumstances he finds. He may, for example, allow unusually higher claims in some categories, such as claims for pensioners, or claims for a particular diagnosis which the physician is specially equipped to treat, or claims for patients covered by the particular fund. He then recommends an adjustment (*Kürzung*) to those parts of the claim which are excessive and cannot be justified. The overview has space for the monitor doctor to write in his recommendations.

All cases in which an adjustment is recommended then go to a monitor committee (*Prüfungsausschuß*). (In some *Länder*, the sickness funds can also initiate a review by the monitor committee.) The committee discusses about 50–80 cases at a sitting, depending on the difficulty of the cases. This volume suggests that the discussions are in fact cursory and that the closest examination is performed by the individual monitor doctor. (Each monitor doctor is given from 20 to 100 cases to work on, depending again on the difficulty of the cases.)

Both the individual doctor to whom the adjustment is applied and the sickness fund have the right to contest the decision of the monitor committee. In the case of such conflict, the monitor committee reconsiders the case once more, in a process called the *"Abhilfverfahren."* The committee has the data on the doctor checked for computation errors and looks for special circumstances of the practice that might have been overlooked the first time. If the committee maintains its decision to apply an adjustment, both the sickness fund and the doctor have the right to appeal the decision to a grievance committee (*Beschwerdeausschuß*). This committee is composed of entirely new doctors. The sickness fund is entitled by law to have at least one nonvoting physician representative on the committee; local AID bylaws may allow more than one such representative, or may allow voting privileges to the fund representatives. In some regions, the doctor in question may be present at the consideration of his case, and in other regions he may only submit written evidence. This committee handles only 7–10 cases per session. Either party—the doctor or the sickness fund—may bring the case before the social court at the regional level; this decision may be appealed to the *Land* social court and ultimately (though this rarely happens) to the Federal Social Court.

Monitoring of drug prescriptions is carried out mostly by the sickness funds. Information about prescriptions is not contained on the claims received by the AIDs. The sickness funds compile average prescription costs per case for each specialty and compare individual physicians' prescription costs with the specialty average. When a large deviation is evident, the funds usually make a motion to bring the case before the monitor committee. Some funds issue a notice of excessive prescriptions to a physician as a first step, and bring the case before the monitor committee only if the excess is continued in the next quarter.

If the monitor committee finds an unjustified excess of prescriptions, it has a range of sanctions available. (These may vary from place to place.) It can put a physician on probation and scrutinize his prescriptions for the next year. It can issue a cutback (called a *Regreß* in the case of drug prescriptions), which is usually only a small percentage (10–15 percent) of the amount deemed excessive. Or, if the committee finds that the physician has prescribed drugs not covered by insurance, it can charge him for the entire cost. If the monitor committee finds no unjustified prescriptions, the sickness fund has the right to appeal the decision to the grievance committee (RVO section 368n).

The Impact of Economic Monitoring

Once the budget constraints on expenditures for physicians' services were removed, collective bargaining over fees and utilization review were the only means by which sickness funds could hope to contain their expenditures. Although the funds shared responsibility with the AIDs for ensuring that the medical services provided to the fund members were sufficient, appropriate, and economical, the actual process of utilization review was left almost entirely in the hands of the AIDs. One result of this division is that data about economic monitoring are almost nonexistent. The AIDs rarely make public any information concerning the number of physicians affected, the amount of money involved in adjustments, or the specific methods used for monitoring. Therefore, any assessment of the impact of economic monitoring is necessarily limited.

Some indication of the importance of economic monitoring might be derived from the number of doctors whose claims are adjusted by it. If only a minute percentage of doctors are affected by adjustments in the monitoring process, monitoring is probably not an important control. Published estimates suggest that anywhere between twenty and seventy percent of physicians are selected for individual monitoring by the monitor committee, but in some areas the figure is as low as five percent.[14] The proportion of physicians whose claims are actually cut back may range from five percent to thirty percent, but is probably closer to the lower end.[15] It is probably safe to conclude that far less than a majority of physicians are affected by economic monitoring but that enough are subjected to cutbacks to make the system more than just a paper tiger.

Another indicator of the significance of economic monitoring might be the amount of money involved. Again, the AIDs keep this information scarce. All available estimates indicate that the amount of money withheld is relatively trivial—averaging anywhere between 0.5 percent and 3.5 percent of the physician's total claims value. In the entire system, the amount of money saved through adjustments is equal to about 0.02 percent of the total claims made by physicians.[16] In the aggregate, the system costs ten times more to administer than it saves in cutbacks, since administrative costs levied by the AIDs are between one and three percent of total payments to physicians, as compared with .02 percent for cutbacks.

Although the economic monitoring system probably has very little financial effect on the individual physician, it may still have a significant deterrent effect. A deterrent effect would be derived from two factors—the certainty of being affected by the monitoring and the severity of the penalties. As to the first criterion, the estimates above suggest that somewhere between five and seventy percent of the physicians are affected, enough to make monitoring a fairly serious concern. Economic monitoring has two types of penalties. The first, the actual cutbacks or claims disallowances, would theoretically have no deterrent effect no matter how large the cutbacks. Since the worst that can happen to a physician is to have some of his claims disallowed, there is in effect no real penalty (or cost) for submitting a large number of excessive claims in the hopes that some of them will be allowed. (Only the cost of paperwork to the individual physician would serve as a restraint on the submission of claims.) There is, however, a second type of penalty. If a physician repeatedly practices uneconomic medicine (as defined by the economic monitor committee), his permit to practice medicine under the public insurance system may be revoked. This would indeed be a serious consequence, since office-based physicians earn approximately eighty-five percent of their income through insurance practice. But this penalty is imposed only after many years of warnings and after appropriate hearings have been granted the physician. In practice, license revocation is extremely rare.[17]

Even if almost no physicians' claims were denied and if the amount of any cutbacks was extremely small, this would not necessarily imply that the monitoring system had no deterrent effect; indeed such evidence might imply that the deterrent effect was so powerful that few physicians ever made any excessive claims. The extent to which physicians "tailor" their practice to fit the norms has not been studied. Some AIDs provide physicians with information on specialty group averages along with the physician's own averages. Others do not provide the individual physicians with the group norms, but physicians whose claims are disallowed or reduced are informed of the relevant norms. It would seem highly likely that the norms would quickly become common knowledge. One recent textbook on the management of insurance practice published a table purporting to tell how often physicians in different specialties could perform a "thorough examination" and still fall within the acceptable limits for their specialty. Accordingly, general practitioners could perform a thorough exam on 25–30 percent of their patients, internists on 40–50 percent, pediatricians on 60–70 percent and gynecologists on 100 percent.[18]

For the income-maximizing physician, a rational strategy under economic monitoring would be to seek to make claims each quarter in an amount just under the upper tolerance limit (e.g., the average plus sixty percent) for each category of service. Such behavior would drive up the averages in the next quarter. If the AIDs were unable to increase the size of the pool they received from the sickness funds, all physicians would receive a lower proportion of their claims, since the ratio of the net divisible pool to the total valid claims would be lowered. But since the pool is now set equal to the amount of total valid claims, this income-maximizing behavior of individual physicians would also lead to a larger collective income for the profession. And even before the switch to fee-for-service determination of the pool, any increase in total claims value generated by such income-maximizing behavior could be used by the AIDs as evidence to support a larger pool in the next round of negotiations.

Unfortunately, it is impossible to test this hypothetical model empirically. One would expect the assumption of income-maximizing behavior to be only partially true, first because physicians' behavior is not purely motivated by income maximization, and second, because the services they *can* perform are circumscribed by the number of patients and kinds of problems that come to them. On the other hand, there are undoubtedly numerous procedures for which the indication is very vague and which can thus be used to "pad" claims.

Overall there is no strong evidence that economic monitoring has much impact on the volume of physicians' services, and many analysts of the health insurance system believe that it has no impact at all. Collectively, physicians have been able to neutralize the system, largely by pressing for more narrowly defined reference groups as the standard of comparison. Through litigation, the process of economic monitoring has become more and more refined, so that AIDs must now consider practice location (e.g., city, suburban, rural), size of practice, and availability of particular diagnostic or therapeutic equipment when they construct a group average as a standard for any individual. With so many variables, the reference groups become extremely small and homogeneous, so that the standards are now sometimes dubbed "mosaic averages."[19]

The possible effectiveness of economic monitoring is severely compromised by the requirement that the reference group used to set a standard must have the same equipment and offer a similar mix of services as the individual physician being monitored.[20] Economic monitoring becomes simply a way of separating physicians into little isolated groups who practice in the same way. And any physician's practice will be found to be "economical," as long as there is some small group of physicians who practice as he does. The economic monitoring system is thus unable to set any constraints on the acquisition of capital equipment by physicians, because each physician has a right to be compared with physicians who have similar equipment. Moreover, because the system has no *outside standards* of appropriate care, derived from some basis other than taking the average of what small groups of physicians do, any small group can create a standard of appropriate care. As a striking example, the apparent excesses in use of X-rays among physicians with radiation equipment (see chapter 6) could not be curtailed by the economic monitoring system, because these physicians can be compared only with other physicians who have similar equipment.

According to one study, about one-quarter of the increase in expenditures for physicians' services can be traced to changes in the mix of services toward more expensive procedures (independent of changes of fee schedule prices of services), and about one-quarter to increases in the number of procedures performed.[21] But economic monitoring, as it is currently conducted, is incapable of constraining either changes in service mix or continuous growth in volume. As long as small groups of physicians alter the mix of services at about the same time, any individual physician will not be subject to monetary cutbacks. And as long as all physicians gradually increase their output of services, each individual can increase his own output under the protection of a constantly rising group average.

The Latent Functions of Economic Monitoring

Since economic monitoring appears to be so ineffectual in the control of expenditures for physicians' services, yet burdens physicians with an enormous amount of paperwork, one wonders what purposes *are* served by the system. Economic monitoring evolved during the period when physicians were paid collectively. Given the fixed sum of money available to each AID, the physicians' incentive was not to keep total costs down but to monitor their own members who might make excessive claims on the pool, to the detriment of all the other doctors in the region. Seen from this vantage point, economic monitoring appears as an orderly and fair way of controlling the intraprofessional distribution of income, when the total income for the profession is fixed.

Two standards are used in the monitoring process to help ensure an equal distribution of income among members of an AID. First, the system of declining marginal fees used by many AIDs helps to lower the income of large practices. And second, the standard used as the main yardstick in the monitoring, i.e., the average per patient claim of all similar doctors in the community, could not be a better one for preventing the development of extremes of wealth within the profession. By using the group averages as the standard against which individual claims are measured, the AID pressures all doctors' incomes toward the mean. To the extent that "extenuating circumstances" are allowed to justify claims outside the normal tolerance range, the standardizing effect of the monitoring is lessened. It is probably not coincidental that physicians have used the courts to introduce more and more "extenuating circumstances" and "special characteristics of the practice" into the monitoring system since the switch to a fee-for-service method of calculating the pool. Now that the pool is not fixed in advance, there is little incentive to control intraprofessional income distribution.

Were data available on income distribution within specialties, one would expect to find less income inequality within any given West German specialty than within its American counterpart, since German physicians' incomes are pushed toward specialty-specific norms. Lacking such data, Lorenz curves for the medical profession as a whole were drawn for the United States and West Germany (See figure 7.1).[22] Income equality is significantly greater among West German office-based physicians than among American physicians in independent practice (the group most like German office-based physicians). Moreover, the curve for the American independent practitioners is based on net income, while the German curve is based on gross income, so the difference in distribution of gross income is presumably even greater than shown, because income taxes tend to equalize the distribution of income. The distribution for American salaried physicians is very close to that for German office-based physicians, suggesting that economic monitoring does indeed have the effect of equalizing income.

One side effect of the statistical methods used in economic monitoring is that specialties with a large number of doctors, a low average claim per case, and a broad range of procedures are disadvantaged, and small groups of physicians with high average claims per case and more homogeneous service mixes are favored.[23] These differential effects occur because the economic monitoring system is based on the assumption of a normal distribution of physicians' average claims around the specialty mean. The more asymmetrical the actual distribution, the greater the

Figure 7.1 Income distribution among Physicians in West Germany and the United States.

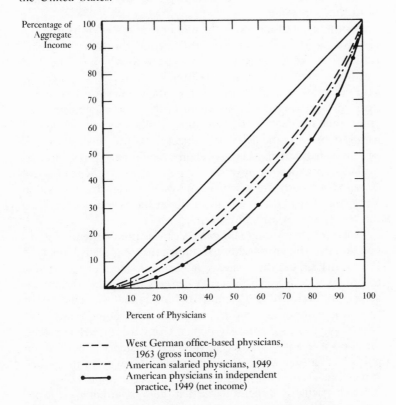

West German office-based physicians, 1963 (gross income)
American salaried physicians, 1949
American physicians in independent practice, 1949 (net income)

Sources: Lange, *Deutsche Ärzteblatt*, 1965, cited in Paul Lüth, *Niederlassung und Praxis* (Stuttgart: Thieme, 1969), p. 110; George Stigler, *Trends in Employment in the Service Industries* (New York: National Bureau of Economic Research, 1956), p. 131.

number of physicians who will be "caught" by the fixed screening criterion. Since primary care specialties and practices are more likely to produce a wide variety of services and to be asymmetrically distributed around the mean, more physicians in these groups will be subject to scrutiny and cutbacks. Also, when the screening criterion (or cutoff point for further scrutiny) is a fixed percentage of the average monetary value of claims, and when the absolute value of the mean is very low, a very small change in the absolute value of an individual physician's mean claim will push him over the limit. Thus, physicians in specialties with a low average claims value will be monitored when their claims exceed the average by a small monetary amount, whereas physicians in specialties with a high average claims value can have a large deviation from the mean in absolute DM, but still not be subjected to further screening.[24]

Another latent function of the monitoring system is its role as a form of symbolic action.[25] Economic monitoring as a symbol conveys two contradictory messages, each of which can be used by the medical profession to bolster its position. Through the very elaborate system of peer review, the medical profession appears to be engaged in controlling health care expenditures by controlling the behavior of its members. When the cost of medical care is debated in the national political arena, the medical organizations can point to their economic monitoring procedures as evidence that they are aggressively policing each other to control costs. When costs are discussed, physicians can draw attention away from fee increases by talking about their careful scrutiny of the "economy" of each physician's practice.

Economic monitoring also gives sickness fund patients the impression that their care is limited, unlike that of private patients.[26] Physicians can use the existence of economic monitoring (regardless of its weakness) to persuade patients that public health insurance is "second class," simply by hinting that the standards of economic monitoring prevent physicians from doing more. And even if physicians vigorously denied that care for sickness fund members is in any way inferior, the sheer existence of controls on publicly financed services would probably convey to the public that public sector health insurance is somehow limited.

It is particularly difficult to see that the standard of average per patient cost has anything to do with economic standards of care. "Economy," in the normal sense of the word, implies finding a relatively inexpensive method of reaching a given goal. In the case of medical care, economy implies comparisons between different treatments for the same disease. The West German monitoring system does not make such comparisons. It makes comparisons only between the incomes of different doctors in the same region. The argument of the AIDs about the effectiveness of economic monitoring thus makes the assumption that those doctors whose incomes (claims) are near the average are also using more economical forms of treatment.

The assumption seems unwarranted. First, there is no reason to believe that the average cost of treating all patients reflects anything about the efficiency or cost of treating a particular patient. A standard of average cost may conceal gross inefficiencies in individual cases.

Second, there is no a priori reason to believe that most doctors in the community practice medicine economically. It is important to note that the system of economic monitoring makes this assumption; at the heart of the system is the belief that most doctors practice "economic" medicine, and that the monitoring system needs only to catch the doctors on the fringes. On the one hand, the system's ostensible purpose is to monitor "economy," but on the other hand, the system itself assumes that most doctors practice economically. In this sense, the monitoring system is designed to protect the status quo, to protect medicine as it is practiced by the majority of doctors. Seen in this context, a monitoring system which used disease-related criteria of care would be a radical innovation, and would probably require radical changes in the way medicine is practiced.

Third, the "average per patient cost" standard is itself derived from the prices assigned to various medical services in the official fee schedules. In effect, the monitoring process translates the relative prices established in the fee schedules into measures of relative "economy." This is another form of protecting the medical practice status quo: average per patient cost (and thus "economy" in medical practice) is determined not by any standard of what works (i.e., outcome measures) but by the price tags assigned to medical procedures in a bargaining process totally separate from the monitoring system.

Economic monitoring, through its use of an average standard of care, also helps protect the status quo practice of medicine in a qualitative sense. It limits innovation, in that it assumes that what most doctors are doing is right, and holds all doctors to those standards. There is, of course, some room for innovation. Presumably, for example, a particularly expensive procedure would not raise the average per patient cost, if it eliminated the need for several less effective and less expensive procedures. Also, new technology is allowed to enter the practice of medicine through the review of special facilities and apparatus that is part of the monitoring system. To the extent that the average cost standard does not govern—i.e., to the extent that extenuating circumstances are allowed to override the deviation from the cost norm as the criterion for claims adjustment—the system does allow for innovation. But it is important to note that innovation by an individual physician is limited only to those circumstances recognized by the monitor committee as justifying factors. Other innovations that might be termed changes in the "style of practice"—for example, emphasizing preventive care or personal counseling—would be hindered by the present system, because physicians would have "excessive" costs in one category of service ("consultations" in this case) relative to their peers.

When government programs provide benefits that are contingent on sickness, proof of illness becomes an event with economic and political implications, as well as medical. In West Germany, where insured workers receive wage continuation payments in the event of illness, the material benefits contingent on illness are substantial. As we have already seen, cash benefits constituted the single largest expenditure of sickness funds in the period before the introduction of the new Law on Wage-Continuation Payments.

In addition to service benefits, German health insurance includes substantial cash benefits in replacement of lost earnings. Until recently, these cash benefits were the source of a major class distinction between social benefits for white-collar and blue-collar workers. Prior to 1957, white-collar (i.e., salaried) workers received wage continuation payments from their employers in the amount of 100 percent of their normal salary, effective from the first day of illness. Blue-collar workers, by contrast, received wage continuation payments totaling only 65 percent of their net earnings, with 60 percent being paid by the sickness funds and 5 percent by the employer; in addition, there was a three-day waiting period (from onset of illness) before the blue-collar worker could collect. If a blue-collar worker remained ill for fourteen or more days, wage continuation payments would be made retroactive to the first day of illness.[1] In 1957, just before the federal elections, the cash benefit program was changed so that blue-collar workers now received 90 percent of their net earnings during illness, with 65–75 percent being paid by the sickness funds and 15–25 percent by the employers.[2] The waiting period was reduced to two days. Most recently, a new law passed in 1969 (effective January 1, 1970) requires most employers to assume the full burden of wage continuation for the first six weeks of a worker's illness.[3]

In order to receive wage continuation payments, a worker must be certified by an insurance doctor as "unable to work." A copy of every sick leave certificate issued by physicians is sent to the relevant sickness fund to inform the fund of the patient's eligibility for wage payments. Insurance doctors thus play an important role in the allocation of cash benefits, since their decisions determine the validity of the insured person's claim to payments, as well as the length of time for which payments may be claimed.

Medical sociologists have long recognized that the decision whether to "be unable to work" is often a discretionary decision by the patient.[4] The West German health insurance program involves a classic instance of the problem of "moral hazard" in insurance.[5] The individual can benefit substantially by claiming insurance benefits, and this incentive incorporated in the insurance program may "tempt" the individual to make decisions (namely, to be "unable to work") which he would not make in the absence of the financial incentive. Moreover, the individual's decision and economic gain flowing from it impose some costs on society, or in this case, on the employer and eventually on other members of the same sickness fund.

Insurance doctors are often caught in a difficult position under this system. On the one hand, the physician is supposed to be a patient advocate in the sense that he is supposed to provide the best care for each patient. His primary interest, both by training and by temperament, is in the health of the patient. On the other hand, his role as "certifier" for cash benefits means that he is also guardian of the public till; physicians determine the volume of claims against employers and the sickness fund treasuries. Insurance doctors are thus expected to reconcile the competing claims of individual patients and the sickness fund administration.

The sickness funds' solution to this dilemma was to hire their own "control doctors" (*Vertrauensärzte*) whose primary loyalty was clearly to the funds. Beginning in the 1920s, the funds began to hire such doctors on a salaried basis. The control doctors had no patient constituency of their own. They could not have a regular ambulatory care practice. Instead, control doctors were paid by the funds to conduct examinations of patients who had been certified as unable to work by their own insurance doctors, with whom the funds had individual contracts but who they had some reason to believe were malingering or otherwise fraudulently collecting cash benefits. The use of control doctors was apparently stimulated by the high rates of unemployment during the 1920s, and the corresponding fears of the sickness fund administrators that members would use their wage continuation payment insurance as a substitute for unemployment benefits.[6] In 1930, what had already become a widespread practice by the funds was incorporated into the Imperial Insurance Code; sickness funds were required by law to conduct "timely monitoring in requisite cases of sick leave certificates as well as prescriptions issued by treating physicians."[7] In 1934, the administrative responsibility for organizing the control doctor service or boards of control doctors (*Vertrauensärztliche Dienst*) was transferred to the pension insurance authorities of each state (*Landesversicherungsanstalt*).

Control doctors are licensed physicians salaried by the state pension authorities. Although they are licensed physicians with the same training as their counterparts in office and hospital practice, they are not allowed to treat patients, but may only perform examinations at the request of sickness funds and recommend certain courses of action (for example, termination of a sick leave certificate, performance of additional diagnostic tests, or initiation of therapeutic procedures). Approximately half of all control doctors are specialists. As of December 1970, there were 1,140 control doctors, with a ratio of one for every 23,661 insured persons, and one for every 45 office-based physicians. The number of control doctors has been declining since World War II, both absolutely and in proportion to the total population. An analysis of the age structure of the board of control doctors over a five-year period demonstrates that younger doctors are not being attracted to the service at a rate sufficient to replace older doctors and staff all the vacant positions (see table 8.1).

Table 8.1 Age Structure of Board of Control Doctors

Age	1966	1971
31–35	.7%	.5%
36–40	4.2	2.3
41–45	22.4	5.3
46–50	29.6	27.3
51–55	21.9	29.6
56–60	15.5	21.9
61–65	4.7	12.5
66+	1.0	.5

Source: Deutscher Bundestag, 6. Wahlperiode, Drucksache VI/3200, p. 142.

In 1970, when the new Law on Wage Continuation Payments went into effect, liability for wage payments during the first six weeks of illness was transferred from the sickness funds to the employers. The transfer of liability to employers had been part of the Social Democratic Party platform for many years. The law became politically possible in 1969 when a sudden and unexpected boom in the economy during 1968 gave employers windfall profits, since their major labor expenses had been set by the collective bargaining contracts between unions and employers during the recession of the previous year. The Social Democratic politicians were able to capitalize on this circumstance and muster enough political support for the new law by presenting it as a means of having employers "pay back" some of their excess profits without having to renegotiate all the collective bargaining contracts.

Employers feared that with the new law, the sickness funds would not have any incentive to monitor certificates very aggressively and that workers would be able to exploit the new system easily. As part of a political compromise in the passage of the bill, two new control mechanisms were introduced to provide an incentive to workers to behave responsibly. First, members of the sickness funds were given a rebate or bonus of DM 10 (about $3.00) for every unused voucher they submitted to the fund, up to a maximum of DM 30 per year. And second, a cost-sharing provision for prescription drugs required all patients to pay twenty percent of each prescription cost, up to a maximum of DM 2.50 (about 80 cents).

Although the major financial burden of wage continuation payments was transferred to employers, the boards of control doctors remained intact. Many reformers would like to transform the board of control doctors from an institution of control, whose only function is to monitor patient and physician behavior, to one that provides and promotes "social medicine." Social medicine in this context is a vague term, but in general means that the control doctors will specialize in problems of rehabilitation and occupational medicine, and that they will incorporate a broader view of medical care that includes an understanding of the patient's relationships to his work, family, and social life. Some data collected by the Ministry of Labor suggest that the behavior of boards of control doctors has changed in some important respects, but that their work still tends to be dominated by a concern for controlling malingering.

To the outside observer, two questions about the board of control doctors are of particular interest. First, one wants to know simply how the institution functions. The board of control doctors stands as an unusual example of a formal mechanism by which society reviews medical decisions that have important nonmedical consequences. Second, one wants to know what the system accomplishes. Does it indeed reverse the decisions of practicing physicians, prevent malingering by patients, and save the sickness funds money? The remainder of this chapter considers these questions.

The monitoring system involves two basic types of decisions: which cases to review, and what constitutes legitimate inability to work. The first type of decision is primarily the responsibility of the sickness funds, although the funds are increasingly relying on both practicing physicians and control doctors to provide advice in the selection of patients for review.[8] The second type of decision is entirely the responsibility of the control doctors.

Before 1969, the Imperial Insurance Code mandated that the sickness funds monitor the inability to work of insured persons and the prescription of benefits "in the cases where requisite." A definition of "requisite" was not provided in the law, and so evolved simply through practice and litigation. The new Law on Wage Continuation Payments changed the Imperial Insurance Code to make the criteria for selection of cases slightly more specific. The RVO now reads that the funds are obligated to seek the recommendation of a control doctor in cases of inability to work where such an examination is necessary "to assure the success of treatment" or "to eliminate reasonable doubts about the inability to work."[9] This new mandate gives the sickness funds authority to use the control doctors to upgrade the quality of care provided its members by allowing the solicitation of second opinions about diagnostic and therapeutic decisions.

Traditionally, decisions about which patients should receive examinations by control doctors were made entirely by the sickness funds. A fund, having received copies of all sick leave certificates written for its members, would decide which members should be required to visit a control doctor and when (i.e., how long after the beginning of the illness). The funds claim that they make such decisions on medical and other criteria which allow them to differentiate cases substantially. Such criteria include: nature and severity of illness, frequency of illness, frequency of change of physician, correspondence between the stated diagnosis and the length of sick leave certified, nature of employment, age of the insured person, and length of membership in the fund. In practice, the selection procedure was apparently not nearly so refined as the funds claim, since in most regions well over eighty percent of all patients certified as sick were actually called in ("summoned") for review by a control doctor.[10] Since the introduction of the new law in 1970, there has been a trend toward more selectivity and away from the "mass summonses" to the control doctors. Surveys conducted by the Ministry of Labor and Social Affairs during September 1970 and February and March 1971 found that only between five and ten percent of all new sick leave certificates were selected by funds to be examined by a control doctor.[11]

Patients, insurance doctors, and employers also have the right to request an examination by a control doctor, but his services are rarely invoked by any party other than the sickness funds (see table 8.2). Even in the period after 1970, when employers were

Table 8.2 Proportion of All Summonses to Board of Control Doctors Requested by Various Parties

| | Type of Patient | | |
Requested by:	Compulsory Member, Blue-Collar	Compulsory Member, White-Collar	Voluntary Member
Employer	4–5%	4–6%	1–2%
Insured person	1–2	1–2	1–3
Treating physician	5–7	19–21	9–22
Sickness fund	86–90	71–76	73–89

Source: Deutscher Bundestag, 6. Wahlperiode, Drucksache VI/3200, appendix B, tables 7–9.

liable for wage continuation payments during the first six weeks of an employee's illness, only about five percent of all examinations by control doctors were initiated by employers. It is interesting to note that physicians are far more likely to request control examinations for white-collar patients than for blue-collar patients.

Despite the dramatic decline in the number of summonses issued since 1970, the sickness funds continue to make selection decisions primarily on the basis of whether a patient is eligible to receive wage continuation payments. A piece of evidence that suggests that this is the major criterion for selection is the timing of the issuance of summonses. In 1966, a study commission estimated that most summonses were issued between seven and ten days after the issuance of a sick leave certificate.[12] At this time (i.e., before 1970) fund members could claim wage continuation payments from the funds after three days of inability to work. A recent study found that during the first half of 1971, more than fifty percent of all examinations by control doctors were performed later than the forty-second day of inability to work.[13] Since the majority of sick leave certificates are for less than six weeks, and since the sickness funds become liable for wage continuation payments on the forty-third day of inability to work, it seems clear that the funds are choosing to review cases primarily when a claim against them is involved (see table 8.3).

Table 8.3 Comparison of Timing of Control Doctor Examinations with Length of Sick Leave Certificates

Timing of Examination (day of illness)[a]	Percent of All Exams	Duration of Inability to Work (days)[b]	Percent of All Sick Leave Certificates
		6 or less	33.3%
1–15	13.4%	7	7.8
		8–9	22.5
16–42	36.1	10–12	18.5
		13–14	6.1
43 or subsequent	50.5	more than 14	11.8

Notes: [a]Based on a survey by Arbeitsgemeinschaft für Gemeinschaftsausgaben der Krankenversicherung of all persons who were *actually* examined by control doctors during the first six months of 1971.
[b]Based on a sample survey of sick leave certificates conducted in June 1970.
Source: Deutscher Bundestag, 6. Wahlperiod, Drucksache VI/3200, pp. 20, 23.

These data all suggest that the sickness funds indeed use the control doctor service as a means of controlling claims for wage continuation payments. There is, however, significant regional variation in the patterns of selection of patients for examination by control doctors, and recently many funds have begun experimenting with new models of administration that give control doctors and office doctors more influence in the selection decisions.

The use of control doctor examinations is one area of the health insurance system in which social class distinctions still persist. Although the Law on Wage Continuation Payments eliminated the last major distinction in benefits between white-collar and blue-collar workers, differential treatment of these two groups by sickness funds is still evident, though not so strong as in the period before 1970. In the years before the new law, fewer than seventeen percent of members of white-collar funds with certificates were asked to come before control doctors, in contrast with approximately seventy percent of workers who were members of other funds.[14] Since blue-collar workers at the time collected wage continuation payments from sickness funds, and white-collar workers collected their payments directly from employers, the different rates of control examinations could be explained by the sickness funds' efforts to protect their own financial status. In the period after 1970, when blue-collar and white-collar workers both receive six weeks of benefits from their employers, the discrepancy between the treatment of the two classes has diminished significantly but is still evident: approximately ten percent of all blue-collar certificates and five percent of all white-collar certificates are selected for review.[15] The different rate of review of blue and white-collar workers persists even within the same sickness fund.

Much of the political debate about the proper role of the board of control doctors centers on the question of what the service actually accomplishes. In theory, its original purpose was to prevent illegitimate and excessive claims against the sickness fund treasuries by screening out cases of malingering. In general, the Federation of German Employers' Unions (BDA) takes the position that the work of control doctors is necessary to prevent malingering by workers, and the Association of German Trade Unions (DGB) takes the position that there is no empirical evidence of malingering.[16] More recently, the various interest groups concerned with health insurance have focused attention on interpreting the effects of the reduction in examinations by control doctors since 1970 on the level of employee absenteeism.

Official statistics show a slight increase in morbidity in 1971 as compared with 1969, but the various groups emphasize different alleged causes of the increase. The Federation of German Employers' Unions claims that the weakening of controls exerted by the sickness funds and the control doctors is responsible for the increase, and that the actual rate of absenteeism is even higher than statistics show. Other groups, including the trade unions, sickness funds, and insurance doctors, emphasize the inadequacies of the procedures by which morbidity is estimated, and thus question whether there has in fact been any real increase since 1970.

Ideally, one would want to assess the effectiveness of control doctors in preventing malingering by examining rates of morbidity and/or absenteeism under different systems of monitoring. Such a study would require sophisticated controls for the major factors (other than the practices of control doctors) that determine morbidity rates, such as age, sex, and income of the population, exposure to contagious diseases and other risks, and level of unemployment. The data currently available certainly do not allow such comparisons to be made. It is impossible to conclude from current data that the changes in use of control doctors since 1970 have had any effect, one way or the other, on the level of malingering in the West German population.

The employers' argument—that the slackening of controls on

malingering since 1970 has caused an increase in absenteeism due to illness—is subject to many criticisms. First, there are many problems with the way morbidity is counted. Official statistics use sick leave certificates as a proxy for morbidity rates. This means that only illnesses of working people, and only those illnesses for which a person is required to obtain a certificate, are counted. Many employers do not require their employees to have a sick leave certificate for short illnesses; hence, the discretionary policies of employers have some influence on morbidity statistics. Also, illnesses and medical problems which do not prevent a person from working are not counted. A second problem with the employers' argument is that it is based on estimates of morbidity for only three years—1969, 1970, and 1971—and thus fails to take account of extraneous factors that might have influenced the morbidity rate. In particular, there is strong evidence that rates of morbidity in Germany vary with rates of unemployment; morbidity tends to increase during periods of economic growth and high employment.[17] The slight increase in morbidity observed between 1969 and 1971 may well be simply a reflection of this general effect of economic trends. Another factor that many observers feel may be responsible for part of the observed increase is a flu epidemic in 1970.

Using morbidity data to demonstrate effects of changes in policy with respect to control doctors is thus inconclusive. The most important deficiency of this approach is that it fails to link the increase in morbidity or absenteeism (i.e., changes in patient behavior) to specific changes in monitoring policy of either the sickness funds or the control doctors. In order to evaluate the effects of the control doctor service on patient behavior, we need first to understand the specific mechanisms by which the monitoring process screens out cases of malingering.

The system of reviewing workers with sick leave certificates includes two mechanisms by which malingerers are induced to return to work. The actual examinations by control doctors may terminate a valid certificate, thus forcing a worker to return to work, or at least cutting off his eligibility for wage continuation payments. Alternatively, a worker who is summoned for an examination by a control doctor may voluntarily choose to return to work before the date of the examination. Figures 8.1 and 8.2 represent the monitoring process schematically and provide estimates of how patients were affected by the process in 1969 and 1971.[18]

Figure 8.1 Monitoring of Sick Leave Certificates, *1969*

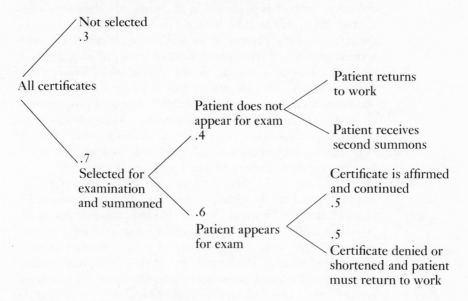

Figure 8.2 Monitoring of Sick Leave Certificates, 1971

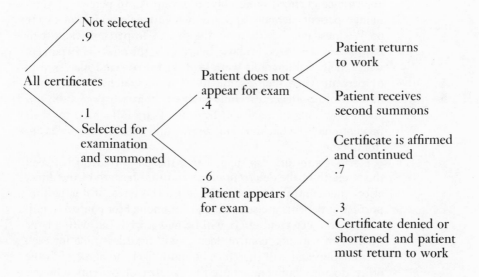

It is apparent from these charts that the monitoring process influences worker behavior, if at all, primarily through its deterrent effect, rather than through the direct examinations. In 1969, about forty percent of all workers with certificates who were summoned did not appear; most of these probably returned to work without a control doctor examination. Only about twenty-one percent of all patients with certificates were examined and found able to return to work. In 1971, when the proportion of all certified workers selected for examination had declined drastically, only about two percent of all workers were actually examined by control doctors and found able to work, and about four percent were summoned but chose not to appear.

Some evidence for the deterrent value of the control doctor system is provided by a study of patients and control doctors by Hans Hartwig.[19] Hartwig suggests that the proportion of workers summoned who actually appear for control doctor examinations will vary with the stringency of control doctors in their decisions whether to affirm certificates. In his study, he examined the records of a board of control doctors that normally examined patients from two different sickness funds, one group (A) on Wednesdays and one group (B) on Fridays. The control doctors worked only half a day on Wednesdays but a full day on Fridays. Their examinations were therefore shorter and less thorough on Wednesdays than on Fridays. Hartwig arranged for the two groups of patients to be switched, so that group A would now be examined on Fridays, and group B on Wednesdays. The rates of appearance changed noticeably: in group A, 56 percent of summoned patients actually appeared when their examinations were on Wednesdays, but the rate dropped to 46 percent when their examinations were on Fridays. In group B, the rate was 59 percent when their examinations were held on Fridays and increased to 61 percent when their examinations were switched to Wednesdays. This evidence certainly suggests that workers' decisions about how long to be absent from work are influenced by their perception of the likelihood of being found able to work by a control doctor.

Hartwig's results also suggest that there is a tradeoff between the strength of the deterrent effect and the strength of the direct effect that control doctor examinations can have. If a large proportion of patients are selected and summoned for control examinations, the deterrent effect will be maximized; but with a large number of patients, control doctors will have less time for each examination and will therefore be more likely to agree with the office doctor's opinion. Thus, the number of patients who are returned to work by decision of the control doctors will be small. If only a small proportion of patients are summoned for control examinations, the deterrent effect will be much smaller, but the examinations will be more thorough and the likelihood of the control doctor's shortening or terminating the certificate will be increased.[20]

The sickness funds use the services of control doctors presumably because they do not think the regular office-based doctors are strict enough in their decisions about patients' inability to work. The control doctor examinations are as much a check on the behavior of physicians as on the behavior of patients. Control doctors are presumably better able to resist patient pressures to grant certificates than office doctors, and thus the control doctors are expected to find cases where office doctors are either co-operating with patients or being deceived by them. A large part of the task of control doctors is also to aid the office doctor in diagnosing and treating vague symptoms and chronic problems that cause repeated absence from work but which the office doctor has been unable to cure effectively.

As with the issue of worker malingering, different groups have different opinions about how "responsible" office physicians are in the granting of certificates. The employers' unions claim that physicians grant certificates too liberally and write them for time periods that are longer than necessary for the given diagnosis. They present as evidence for this claim the fact that many workers return to work before the expiration of their certificates. The sickness funds, on the other hand, claim that physicians underestimate the duration of inability to work so that their patients will have to return and the physicians can earn extra fees by writing a second and third certificate.[21]

No study has collected appropriate data to evaluate these claims satisfactorily. The AIDs do not collect information on physicians' certification behavior as part of their economic monitoring procedures. Although the sickness funds use some norms that relate specific diagnoses to permissible lengths of inability to work, their norms are not universally accepted either by the control doctors or by the insurance doctors. So there is no yardstick by which to measure the correctness of physicians' decisions about illness certificates.

Some indication of the effectiveness of the board of control doctors in controlling or influencing the certification process is given by the proportion of cases in which control doctors contradict the opinions of office physicians. If control doctors are not willing to overturn the certificates issued by other physicians, the

Table 8.4 Proportion of Examinations by Control Doctors in Which Office Doctor's Opinion Was Sustained

	Type of Patient					
	Compulsory Members, Blue-Collar		Compulsory Members, White-Collar		Voluntary Members	
Year	Male	Female	Male	Female	Male	Female
1970	59%	60%	75%	66%	78%	74%
1971	61%	59%	76%	68%	75%	76%

Source: Deutscher Bundestag, 6. Wahlperiode, Drucksache VI/3200, p. 32.

system would clearly not work. One study determined that control doctors found patients with certificates immediately able to return to work in 7 percent of all cases for the nation as a whole, and the rate varied from about 2.3 percent to about 18.7 percent in different regions.[22] Table 8.4 suggests that willingness of control doctors to contradict decisions of office doctors is at least partially influenced by the social class of the patient involved. In general, control doctors are more likely to agree with the patient's own physician if the patient is a white-collar worker than if he is a blue-collar worker, white-collar male than white-collar female, and voluntarily insured than compulsorily insured. It is extremely difficult to interpret these results; on the one hand, they may mean that blue-collar workers, white-collar females, and compulsory members are more successful at persuading their physicians to write unnecessary certificates for unnecessarily long periods of time. Or they may mean that the control doctors are more sympathetic to the claims of high-income white-collar workers, and especially white-collar males, that they are in fact unable to work.

Control doctors may disagree with office physicians in two ways. They may find that a sick leave certificate is entirely unwarranted, in which case they determine that the patient is immediately able to return to work. Alternatively, they may find that the patient is indeed unable to work, but disagree with the office physician about the length of absence from work that is necessary. The Ministry of Labor study cited above found that each of these reasons accounted for approximately half of the cases in which control doctors did not sustain the decision of the office doctor.[23]

It is difficult to assess whether the decisions of control doctors have any real effect on the level of justified absenteeism. Although the control doctors do not always sustain the decisions of office doctors, office doctors may have learned to accommodate themselves to the norms of control doctors in some ways. They may, for example, be overestimating the amount of time a patient needs for recovery, knowing that the control doctors in their region always cut back the certificates by a certain number of days. From a familiarity with the norms of the control doctors, they may be writing down a diagnosis that justifies the length of certificate they wish to write, rather than the diagnosis they believe to be true. Although there are criminal penalties for this kind of fraud, there are undoubtedly many instances of legitimate doubt where a physician could write down the more serious of two suspected diagnoses, although the evidence for the less serious might be stronger.

Finally, it is impossible to judge whether the control doctor service actually saves the sickness funds and employers money. To answer this question, one would need to do a controlled experiment in which groups of insured persons were matched for income (and therefore income replacement needs) and actual morbidity experience. Nevertheless, regardless of its actual effects, the service undoubtedly has an important symbolic value. The board of control doctors is an institution that symbolically represents the public interest and defends the collective treasury against the private claims of patients and their physicians.

The board of control doctors as an institution is also symbolically important in another sense. The issue of wage continuation payments has always divided the country fairly clearly along class lines. Not only were white-collar and blue-collar workers treated differently as an object of policy, but also attitudes toward reform of wage continuation policy have been sharply divided between labor (employees and their unions) and capital (employers and their unions). Debates about the wage continuation policy are versions of the broader issue of income distribution within the society. Wage continuation amounts to income redistribution in that it distributes income on the basis of some principle other than as a reward for productive labor. The use of illness as the criterion, and consequent displacement of decisionmaking onto physicians, can be seen as an effort to depoliticize income redistribution by making the decisions appear "scientific," "neutral," and "objective."

The foregoing analysis of the board of control doctors suggests that political conflicts are not easily resolved by surrounding small discretionary allocative decisions with the aura of scientific neutrality. The very existence of the board of control doctors signifies that some conflict persists and that there is significant mistrust of the office physicians' decisions. The differential rates of summonses for blue-collar and white-collar workers indicate that the sickness funds tend to use the control doctors as an instrument of differential treatment of different social classes. And the differential rates of sustaining the office physicians' certificates illustrated in table 8.6 certainly suggest that physicians' decisions (either control doctors or office doctors or both) are not class neutral.

Some of the financing and reimbursement methods used in West Germany are similar to cost control strategies that are used or have been advocated in the United States. How well have these mechanisms worked in West Germany? What has been the experience with medical care expenditure growth? And how have cost control mechanisms fared politically?

The West German system has had a combination of four methods of cost control, though these have not always operated continuously, even since 1932. The first method is a legislative *ceiling on permissible tax rates* charged by the sickness funds. In theory, such a ceiling should limit the total revenues available for health services. As we saw in chapter 4, as soon as the funds switched over to a fee-for-service method of calculating the pool, the federal government apparently gave up trying to enforce any legislatively set ceiling. Ceilings on permissible tax rates are very similar to regulation of premiums by state insurance commissions in the United States, and to setting of Medicare premiums by the federal government. In all of these cases, ceilings as a method of cost control can only be as effective as the legislative determination to enforce them.

A second cost control mechanism in the West German system is *prospective negotiation of fixed pools* to cover the costs of office-based physicians' services. Reimbursement from a prospectively negotiated fixed pool is similar to various fixed budgeting strategies used or advocated in the United States, such as health maintenance organizations and foundations for medical care. As we have already seen, sickness funds in West Germany abandoned the method of capitation-based pools set in advance, and now pay the AIDs a pool that is retroactively determined using a fee-for-service method.

The third cost control feature of the West German system is *collective bargaining over the level of physicians' fees*. Sickness funds negotiate with physicians' organizations over both the relative value of various medical procedures and the conversion factors used to determine the actual monetary prices of procedures in a given time period. Collective bargaining over fee levels has been advocated by the Health Care Financing Administration in the United States as a method of determining physicians' fees for Medicaid and Medicare services. In addition, some physicians' unions in the United States have also advocated collective bargaining as the most fair way to determine physicians' fees.

Finally, economic monitoring is a form of *utilization review* that is intended to control health expenditures by exerting downward pressure on the volume of services provided by physicians. Physicians' services are reviewed by their peers to determine whether their practice patterns conform to some general standards of appropriateness and economy. In the United States, utilization review has been used very widely and has been formalized into a government mandated system for review of all hospital services (known as professional standards review organizations) financed by the federal government.

Indicators of Professional Power

Health Expenditure Growth. One measure of health expenditure growth that is of concern in the United States is the proportion of gross national product (GNP) devoted to health care expenditures, or "relative health expenditures." Changes in this measure over time indicate the extent to which national resources are being shifted toward the production of health services and away from other kinds of goods and services (or possibly vice versa).

Cross-national comparisons of health expenditures and growth rates can be suggestive, but not very conclusive. Health expenditures are defined differently in different countries, and data are usually collected in categories that are administratively useful within a particular country's health system. The West German government, for example, does not regularly collect or publish data on all health expenditures; expenditures through the public health system are well documented, but other expenditures (i.e., direct private payments, payments through private health insurance, and payments by other social insurance carriers, such as the pension fund) are difficult to determine.

There have been many attempts to develop comparative estimates of total health expenditures as a proportion of GNP for different countries (see table 9.1), but since each of these depends on making adjustments to account for different national definitions, the estimates should be taken only as very rough. What does emerge is that until recently West Germany was consistently in the middle of the range of relative health expenditures for advanced industrial countries. But by 1975, West Germany led the major Western countries in relative health expenditures.

By almost any indicator, health expenditures in West Germany went virtually out of control during the early 1970s (see table 9.2). From 1960 to 1970, total expenditures of the public health system grew at an average annual rate of about 10 percent, but between 1970 and 1975, expenditures grew at nearly double that rate (19.4

Table 9.1 Total Expenditures for Health Services as Percent of Gross National Product for Selected Countries

Country	1960	1970	1975
West Germany	4.4	6.1	9.7
Australia	5.0	5.6	7.0
Canada	5.6	7.1	7.1
France	5.0	6.6	8.1
Netherlands		6.3	8.6
Sweden	3.5	7.5	8.7
United Kingdom	3.8	4.9	5.6
United States	5.3	7.2	8.4
Finland	4.2	5.9	6.8

Source: Joseph G. Simanis and John R. Coleman, "Health Care Expenditures in Nine Industrialized Countries, 1960–76," *Social Security Bulletin* 43 (January 1980): 5.

Table 9.2 Indicators of Cost Control in Statutory Health Insurance (SHI)

Year	Total Expenditures of SHI (million DM)	Annual % Change	SHI as % of GNP	Annual % Change in GNP	Annual % Change in Avg. Wage/ Salary
1960	9,513		3.1		
1961	10,674	+12.2	3.2	+10.0	+10.4
1962	11,947	+11.9	3.3	+8.3	+9.0
1963	12,878	+7.8	3.4	+6.6	+6.2
1964	13,838	+7.5	3.3	+9.6	+9.0
1965	15,786	+14.1	3.4	+9.4	+9.1
1966	18,362	+16.3	3.7	+6.6	+7.3
1967	19,236	+4.8	3.9	+1.0	+3.2
1968	21,513	+11.8	4.0	+9.0	+6.3
1969	28,899	+11.1	3.9	+12.1	+9.2
1970	25,179	+5.4	3.7	+13.3	+14.8
1971	31,140	+23.7	4.1	+11.1	+11.7
1972	36,401	+16.9	4.4	+9.5	+9.0
1973	43,365	+19.1	4.7	+11.2	+11.9
1974	51,809	+19.5	5.2	+7.4	+11.4
1975	60,990	+17.7	5.8	+4.8	+7.0
1976	66,563	+9.1	6.0	+8.9	+7.5

Source: Angaben des Bundesministerium für Arbeit und Sozialordnung, June 13, 1977.

percent). This difference remains even when changes in the number of funds are considered. Expenditures per member grew just under 9 percent per year from 1960 to 1970, but 17.2 percent per year from 1970 to 1975.[1] For the entire period from 1960 to 1975, health care expenditures grew much more rapidly than the gross national product and the average wage and salary. (The one exception—the year 1970—was the year in which employer liability for wage continuation payments began, so that sickness funds experienced a sudden reduction in their payment of cash benefits.) Beginning in 1975, the rate of growth of expenditures began to decrease (see table 9.2).

If health expenditures grew extremely rapidly in West Germany during the 1970s, comparative statistics indicate that it was not alone. In France, health expenditures grew about 17 percent per year between 1970 and 1976. In Sweden, they tripled between 1966 and 1976.[2] In the United States, they grew at an average annual rate of 11.4 percent between 1970 and 1975.[3] Thus it seems that many advanced industrial countries experienced rapid increases in health expenditures. But the fact remains that while West Germany was not unique, whatever cost control mechanisms were built into its national health insurance system did not insulate it from the trend.

Physicians' Share of Health Expenditures. Expenditures for health services in West Germany are growing at a rapid rate, and they are consuming an ever-increasing share of the GNP. Thus, health care providers in general are experiencing a redistribution of income in their favor. If the reimbursement methods described above have any restraining influence at all, they should be most effective in controlling expenditures for ambulatory physicians' services. Examination of the relative shares of sickness fund expenditures going to different types of providers over a long period of time shows that physicians in the ambulatory sector have managed to hold their own quite well against other claims on the sickness fund monies (see table 9.3).

Several significant trends are evident. First, the increasing importance of medical service benefits rather than cash benefits as the major function of social insurance is demonstrated by the decline of cash benefits from almost half of sickness fund expenditures at the beginning of national health insurance to less than ten percent since 1970. Second, the hospitals have been the primary beneficiaries of increased expenditures since the inception of the program; it is important to notice that the category "physi-

Table 9.3 West Germany: Expenditures of Sickness Funds for Selected Categories, as Percent of Total Fund Expenditures

Year	Physicians' Services (office-based)	Drugs and Appliances	Hospital Services	Cash Benefits
1885	17.3	14.0	8.9	45.3
1890	18.2	15.9	10.0	43.5
1895	19.9	15.9	11.4	40.1
1900	19.4	15.1	11.7	41.1
1905	20.4	13.6	12.4	40.3
1910	21.0	13.4	13.7	38.1
1914	22.5	11.5	13.5	35.8
1924	23.5	10.3	13.0	32.8
1930	21.9	11.5	15.6	28.3
1935	23.4	11.8	17.4	21.4
1950	20.1	15.9	19.2	20.6
1955	22.3	15.8	17.8	21.7
1960	19.7	13.7	16.5	28.3
1965	20.2	15.2	18.7	23.4
1970	21.7	19.5	23.9	9.8
1975	18.5	18.8	28.7	7.6

Sources: 1885–1935: J. Hadrich, *Arzthonorar und Morbidität in der sozialen Krankenversicherung* (Berlin: Duncker und Humblot, 1957), p. 50. 1950–65: *Statistisches Jahrbuch der Kassenärztlichen Bundesvereinigung, 1971,* table 26. 1970–75: Bundesministerium für Arbeit und Sozialordung, "Statistische Daten zur konzertierten Aktion im Gesundheitswesen," Bonn, February 28, 1978, mimeo, table 11.

cians' services" in the German data includes only payments to office-based physicians, and that the salaries of hospital physicians are buried in the category "hospital services."

If cash benefits are excluded from total sickness fund expenditures, so as to make the German data more comparable with the United States data in table 9.4, German physicians still appear to have done very well (see table 9.5). From 1885 to 1935, office-based physicians maintained a constant share of about one-third of health service expenditures. Moreover, office-based physicians alone in West Germany receive about the same share of health expenditures as all physicians in the United States—around twenty percent. The comparison is not strictly valid, since in West Germany only health expenditures through the public health insurance system are counted, yet there are significant expenditures outside the public health insurance system. One study of total expenditures in West Germany estimates that in 1976, office-based practices absorbed 17.3 percent of all health

Table 9.4 United States: Health Care Expenditures for Selected Categories, as Percent of Total Expenditures

Fiscal Year	Physicians' Services	Hospital Services	Drugs
1929	27.7	18.1	16.7
1935	26.2	25.7	16.5
1940	24.5	25.1	16.2
1950	22.4	30.7	13.7
1955	21.3	32.8	13.2
1960	21.6	32.9	13.9
1965	21.6	33.8	11.9
1970	19.8	38.0	10.4
1975	19.3	39.1	8.4

Sources: 1929–70: Barbara S. Cooper, Nancy L. Worthington, and Paula A. Piro, "National Health Expenditures, 1929–73," *Social Security Bulletin* 37 (February 1974), p. 12. 1975: Robert M. Gibson and Charles R. Fisher, "National Health Expenditures, Fiscal Year 1977," *Social Security Bulletin* 41 (1978), p. 15.

expenditures, and net earnings of office-based physicians accounted for about 13.5 percent of all expenditures.[4] Thus, even when expenditures outside of the health insurance system are taken into account, the share going to office-based physicians remains very high.

Between 1935 and 1975, the share of fund expenditures going to office-based physicians declined substantially (from almost one-third to about one-fifth). Nevertheless, the fact that office-based physicians receive even one-fifth of expenditures is remarkable, considering the tremendous growth of hospital-based technology since 1935 and the tremendous migration of West German physicians into the hospital sector. In 1976, office-based physicians comprised about 47 percent and hospital-based physicians about 45 percent of the medical profession (see table 4.3). In that year, about 20 percent of sickness fund expenditures went to office-based physicians, and about 31 percent went for *all* hospital care, including the costs of physicians' salaries, wages and salaries of other personnel, and all operating costs of hospitals.[5] Even if one imputes a generous half of all sickness fund expenditures for hospital services to hospital-based physicians, their share is still significantly less than that of office-based physicians.

These figures graphically illustrate the political success of office-based physicians in capturing and protecting a market for themselves. Despite the greater increase of hospital-based physicians and the growth of hospital-based technology over a long

Table 9.5 Physicians' Share of Health Expenditures, U.S. and Germany

Year	Germany[a]	U.S.[b]
1885	31.6%	
1890	32.1	
1895	33.1	
1900	32.9	
1905	34.2	
1910	34.0	
1914	35.0	
1924	35.0	
1929	31.0	27.7%
1930	30.5	
1935	29.8	26.2
1940		24.5
1950	25.3	22.4
1955	28.5	21.3
1960	27.5	21.6
1965	26.3	21.6
1970	24.0	19.8
1975	20.0	19.3

Notes: [a] Office-based physicians' share of sickness fund expenditures, excluding wage continuation payments. [b] All physicians' share of all health expenditures.
Source: Calculated from tables 9.3 and 9.4.

period of time, office-based physicians have held onto an enviable share of health expenditures. That physicians receive a larger share of sickness fund expenditures (about 20 percent) than of all expenditures (about 17 percent) suggests that office-based physicians are actually better able to manipulate the sickness fund system than the private market (i.e., out-of-pocket payments and private insurance payments.)

Physicians' Income. The strength of the office-based sector is further manifested in the incomes of physicians. Office-based physicians in West Germany earn more money on average than nonsalaried physicians in the United States—about $68,000 per year as compared with $58,000 per year in 1975.[6] They also enjoy higher incomes relative to the average wages within their own society: West German office-based physicians earn on the average 6.7 times as much as the average industrial worker, while for

Table 9.6 Income of Physicians in West Germany by Sector

Sector	Income per Physician
Office-based (1971)	DM 113,543[a]
Hospital-based (1972)	
Chiefs of staff	DM 100,000–180,000[b]
Associate physicians (Oberärzte)	DM 48,000–60,000[c]
Staff physicians (Assistenzärzte)	DM 30,000–42,000[c]

Notes: [a]mean net income before taxes, but after deduction of practice costs. [b]net income from hospital services only, before taxes. [c]gross income.

Source: Gesellschaft für Sozialen Fortschritt, *Der Wandel der Stellung des Arztes im Einkommensgefüge* (Bonn, 1974), p. 21.

American physicians the figures is only (!) 5.3 times as much.[7]

Office-based physicians in West Germany also earn significantly more than hospital-based physicians, except for the chiefs of staff who may conduct private office practices. Unfortunately, there are no systematic and periodic surveys of hospital-based physicians, as there are of office-based practices, so that only a rough comparison is possible (see table 9.6). The data on hospital physicians are from the German Hospital Association, and because they do not include income from a variety of outside sources, they probably underestimate the income of hospital-based physicians.[8] Nevertheless, if the mean net income of office-based physicians is nearly double the highest gross income of associate physicians, and almost triple the highest gross income of staff physicians, then office-based practice is certainly much more lucrative than hospital medicine, even by these rough estimates.

As in the United States, there is significant variation in the income of different specialties. Table 9.7 shows the income of different office-based specialists in West Germany in 1971 and 1975. Physicians in specialties that use a great deal of laboratory, radiological, or other mechanical equipment tend to rank higher than physicians who provide relatively time-intensive services (general practitioners, pediatricians, ear-nose-and-throat physicians). Radiologists are consistently at the top.

Table 9.8 presents a comparison of the incomes of some specialties in the United States and West Germany. These comparisons are very crude, however, and should be taken as only suggestive, since the data are for office-based physicians only in West Germany and all physicians in the United States. Also,

Table 9.7 Mean Net Income of Physicians by Specialty in West Germany, 1971–75

Specialty	1971		1975	
	DM	Index[a]	DM	Index[a]
All physicians	113,543	100.0	149,247	100.0
Nonspecialists	102,958	90.7	135,123	90.5
Internists	136,322	120.0	180,953	121.2
OB-GYN	112,659	99.2	160,078	107.2
Pediatrics	90,704	79.8	116,356	78.0
Ophthalmology	144,941	127.6	186,333	124.8
ENT	118,643	104.4	130,982	87.8
Orthopedics	136,370	120.1	180,989	121.3
Surgery	120,384	106.0	131,866	88.4
Dermatology	70,698	62.2	147,161	98.6
Radiology	177,582	156.4	269,228	180.4
Lung specialists	107,767	94.9	122,015	81.8
Urology			173,549	116.3
Neurology	103,399	91.0	144,648	96.9
Group practices			137,648	92.2

Notes: [a]"Mean net income" is gross income minus practice costs, before taxes. "Nonspecialists" includes general practitioners and specialists in general medicine. The index shows the ratio of the specialty mean to the mean for all physicians.
Source: Ulrich Geissler, Beratungsunterlage No. 1066: Ergebnisse der "Kostenstrukturerhebung für ärztliche und zahnärztliche Praxen 1975" des Statistischen Bundesamtes, Bundesverband der Ortskrankenkasse, Bad Godesberg, 14 September 1977, mimeo, p. 10. Indexes calculated by author.

Table 9.8 Physician Mean Net Incomes: U.S. and West Germany, 1975

Specialty	United States		West Germany	
	$	Index	DM	Index
All specialties	56,361	100.0	149,247	100.0
General practice	45,410	80.6	135,123	90.5
Internal medicine	56,982	101.1	180,953	121.2
Surgery	68,226	121.1	131,866	88.3
Pediatrics	44,250	78.5	116,356	78.0
OB-GYN	63,316	112.3	160,078	107.3
Radiology	75,239	133.5	269,228	180.4

Note: U.S. figures represent mean net income per physician (all physicians); West German figures represent mean net income per office-based physician.
Sources: West Germany: Table 9.7 United States: American Medical Association, *Profile of Medical Practice 1978* (Chicago, 1978), pp. 246 and 247.

"surgery" for the United States includes ophthalmologists and urologists, who are not included in the German "surgery" category. In both countries, pediatricians and general practitioners earn below average incomes, though general practitioners do slightly better in West Germany. Internists earn significantly above the mean physician income in West Germany, while in the United States they earn about the mean. The most striking difference is for radiologists, who earn about eighty percent more than the physician average in West Germany but only about thirty-three percent more in the United States.

In view of the tremendous growth in health expenditures, the ability of office-based physicians to maintain a relatively constant share of the expenditures despite increases in hospital-based technology and shifts of physicians into the hospital sector, and the extremely high income enjoyed by office-based physicians, it is difficult to avoid the conclusion that the sickness funds have been a rather ineffective countervailing power to the AIDs. Some reasons for their weakness have been hinted at in chapter 5. A more thorough analysis of their power position is now warranted.

Reasons for the Weakness of Sickness Funds

There are many theories about the factors that compromise the power position of the sickness funds relative to the AIDs. The most common argument is that the AIDs are more concentrated than the funds. While there are only about seventeen AIDs (one in each *Land* or independent city), there are about fourteen hundred sickness funds. According to this theory, the AIDs use a strategy of "divide and conquer"; they favor numerous negotiations with separate funds because they play the funds off against each other. Many people believe that if the sickness funds could centralize their fee negotiations more, they would be in a stronger position.[9]

The appealing logic of this argument is contradicted by the experience of the funds that do conduct fee negotiations exclusively at the federal level. AID contracts with the various public employee plans (i.e., Ministries of Defense, Interior, and Labor) and with the substitute funds stipulate fee levels far above those negotiated by the RVO funds. In 1973 and 1974, fees in non–RVO fund contracts ranged from 60 to 80 percent higher than fees in RVO fund contracts.[10] Thus, centralization of fee negotiations by itself is not necessarily a cure for sickness fund problems.

The driving force in the system is competition *among* the funds. The different sets of funds have differing financial strengths, owing to the different tax rates, risk mixes, and levels of taxable income of their members. Yet there is a strong drive for the funds to offer the same levels of health services. The RVO sickness funds in particular are constantly running from the popular charge that they provide second-class medicine. Physicians can wield a great deal of influence in shaping public demand for higher fees and greater benefits in the RVO system, simply by hinting to their RVO patients that the low payment levels and benefit coverage of RVO funds prevent patients from getting care that would be given to substitute fund or private patients.

Given the deep-rooted cultural belief that everyone should have access to any medical services necessary to preserve good health, and the legal entitlement to all care that is "necessary and effective," all of the sickness funds are constrained to upgrade their benefits to cover the expanding scope of services deemed "necessary and effective." But there is no objective definition of "necessary and effective." Rather, whatever physicians customarily do in a given clinical situation becomes the norm for that situation. The hierarchical system of sickness funds then generates a "trickle down" of customary standards. Physicians first begin to provide a particular service (say, a new diagnostic test) to private patients. The substitute funds, in order not to lose members to private insurance companies, must offer to cover the same service. At this point, if there is a discrepancy between services the private and substitute fund patients receive and those the RVO fund patients receive, pressure will be put on the RVO funds. One way this happens is that popular pressure forces legislators to declare the new service a mandatory benefit. The more usual mechanism is that a patient or *Land* or local welfare agency litigates the right of a sickness fund to refuse to pay for some service. By and large, the courts have played an expansionist role.[11] Since the RVO guarantees patients care that is "sufficient and effective according to the standards of medical practice," the standard of care provided to private and substitute fund patients naturally becomes the standard that courts use for RVO funds.

Competition among the different types of funds explains the source of pressure on sickness funds constantly to expand their coverage and benefit levels. The sickness funds actually have very little leverage in influencing their own expenditure levels. Through collective bargaining, the funds can exercise some control over the fees for individual services. But even assuming that they could tightly control both the relative value scale and the conversion factors, they would still need to control other key determinants of their expenditures—the number of insured persons, the incidence of illness or injury among the insured population, and the number and mix of services performed and prescribed per patient. And as we saw in chapter 7, the system of economic monitoring gives sickness funds very little leverage over the number and mix of services, because the funds' representation on monitor committees is very weak, and because the use of "average claims value" as a norm does not impose any outside standards on physician practice patterns.

The two instruments for setting limits on the aggregate payments to physicians have both been eliminated. One, the modified capitation formula for prospectively setting the size of the pool, was abandoned voluntarily by a few sickness funds at first. Then a combination of pressure from physicians and popular sentiment against different payment mechanisms in the public and private plans led to a complete switch to the fee-for-service method of determining the pool.

The statutory limit on the tax rate of sickness funds might have served as a second line of defense against cost escalation. But legislators naturally followed the incentives of elected politicians. They expanded benefit coverage in the public insurance program, thus providing small benefits to a large number of constituents, and financed the expansion by allowing the tax rate on the wage base to rise, and eventually, in 1971, allowing the wage base to rise automatically.

Reasertion of the Limits on Collective Power

By 1975, the runaway growth of health insurance expenditures had become a topic of major public concern. The federal government, which for many years had promoted expansions in benefit coverage while allowing the erosion of cost control mechanisms, was suddenly more concerned with assuring the fiscal solvency of the entire social security system, and particularly the pension scheme. But legislators and ministry officials found a dearth of information about costs and expenditures in the health insurance system. In the early 1970s, two major studies helped rectify the information deficiency. The Society for Social Progress conducted the first major study of physicians' incomes, whose results were then given major play in the popular press. And the Ministry of Labor appointed the Expert Commission on Health Insurance Reform, which examined the internal workings of the health insurance system and its control mechanisms.

Physicians, of course, opposed any cost control mechanisms, but when faced with strong determination on the part of the government to tackle the cost problem, adopted the strategy of "voluntary controls" to stave off more stringent mandatory controls. In 1976, the Federal Association of Insurance Doctors concluded voluntary agreements with the federal associations of local, factory, guild, and agricultural funds to limit spending for ambulatory care.[12] The contract placed an eight percent ceiling on annual growth of expenditures for services of office-based physicians—a significant restraint in comparison to the annual average growth rates of thirteen to fourteen percent in the two preceding years.[13]

By this time, however, there was consensus among government officials, sickness fund administrators, trade union leaders, and employers that the public health insurance system had serious structural weaknesses, and in 1977, Parliament passed a major piece of reform legislation, the Health Care Cost Containment Act (HCCCA).[14] The legislation was aimed at the two main problems identified above—the competitive dynamic among sickness fund types, and the lack of direct controls on the total volume of sickness fund expenditures.

The HCCCA introduces two measures to equalize the financial strength of the sickness funds. First, there will be some redistribution of cost among sickness funds of the same type (i.e., local, factory, and so on). The ratio of expenditures to total taxable wage base ("need quotient") will be computed for each sickness fund, and if a particular fund's ratio exceeds the average ratio for that type of fund, a financial redistribution will be undertaken by the state authorities. To make sure that this general risk pooling does not undermine cost control incentives of individual funds, the need quotient will include only expenditures for services mandated by Parliament. This type of equalization is voluntary and has so far occurred in only one *Land*.

Second, some equalization of the costs of medical care for pensioners will occur through an extra tax levied on all members of public health insurance. Unlike the general equalization, which uses norms specific to each type of fund, and therefore preserves the major differences among fund types, the extra costs for pensioners' health care will be spread uniformly among the sickness funds. These two measures essentially move the system of financing of public health insurance more toward community rating. The sickness funds will still operate as administratively autonomous entities, but some of their fiscal autonomy will be reduced by the broader spreading of risks.

The HCCCA also mandates development of a single, nation-wide relative value scale for all sickness funds, to replace the separate ones currently used by the RVO and substitute funds. The sickness funds will still be able to negotiate different conversion factors, so that the substitute funds will presumably still pay physicians higher fees. But the consolidation of negotiations over the relative value scale is intended to strengthen the ability of sickness funds to reorient priorities in service delivery through a differential reward structure.

The major instrument of the HCCCA is the requirement for a prospectively negotiated ceiling on expenditures for certain health services. These ceilings are in a sense an attempt to restore the old capitation-based pools negotiated in advance. The HCCCA calls for three separate expenditure ceilings, for physicians' services, dentists' services, and prescription drugs.

The new ceilings differ from the old system of setting the pool in several important ways, but the principle of fixed budgeting is the same. Under the old (pre-1955) payment method, the size of the pool was pegged primarily to the number of patients insured by the sickness fund. Under the new legislation, the size of the pool (actually, the rate of growth of the pool) is tied to broader economic indicators—the average wage base of the sickness funds, the average wage or salary of all employed persons, and costs of medical practice. The old system was never strictly a capitation system, nor is the new system strictly tied by a fixed formula to economic indicators. But the ceilings do exert pressure on physicians as a group to constrain the volume of services, and they relate physicians' income to the income of other members of society.

Another major difference between the new ceilings and the old method of setting the pool is that negotiations on the expenditure ceilings are now highly centralized. Whereas earlier each sickness fund could negotiate individually with the respective AID over the size of the total pool, the new expenditure ceilings are established by a single national commission, the Concerted Action on Health Affairs. The "concerted action" is a conflict resolution device that is also used in other areas of German policymaking, most notably labor-management conflicts. A concerted action is a large group of representatives of all parties affected by an issue which seeks to resolve conflicts through discussion and consensus. Though it is a formally constituted body, its procedures are less formalized than collective bargaining or compulsory arbitration.[15] A similar institution in the United States is the Health Insurance Benefits Advisory Committee (HIBAC) that was created by the Social Security Administration to help implement Medicare and Medicaid.

The Concerted Action on Health Affairs consists of about sixty representatives of sickness funds, physicians, dentists, pharmaceutical manufacturers, apothecaries, hospitals, trade unions, employer unions, and federal, state, and municipal governments, and is empowered to promulgate yearly expenditure ceilings. Should the Concerted Action fail to come to an agreement on ceilings for physicians' (or dentists') services, the Federal Association of Insurance Doctors (or of Insurance Dentists) is required to negotiate a ceiling directly with the Federal Association of Sickness Funds. As a final fail-safe, if an agreement still cannot be reached, then an expenditure ceiling will be created through compulsory arbitration.

Once the ceilings on expenditures for physicians' and dentists' services have been set, the sickness funds and AIDs are required to abide by the ceilings in their negotiations on the size of the pool. Any increases which are negotiated at any level (federal, state, or county) must be consistent with the national guidelines. If physicians (or dentists) provide more services than can be covered by the pool, their individual reimbursements will be cut back uniformly. (For example, if the total fee schedule value of all physician claims in a given quarter is 125% of the value of the negotiated pool, all physicians will be reimbursed at 80% of the fee schedule rate for every service.)

The new ceilings on expenditure growth essentially serve the same function as the old prospectively negotiated pools. And they restore the old "quotient" system under which the AID distributes the pool on a fee-for-service basis, but only in proportion to the ratio of total pool to total claims. The HCCCA centralizes negotiations at the national level—a move which might strengthen the hand of sickness funds. But the expansion of participants to include representatives from all organizations concerned with health insurance will surely dilute the ability of the Concerted Action to reach decisive agreements. In fact, the use of a concerted action as the bargaining forum instead of direct negotiations between the Federal Association of Insurance Doctors (or Dentists) and the Federal Association of Sickness Funds was a compromise that the labor ministry was forced to accept to assure passage of the bill.

The Health Care Cost Containment Act also takes steps to strengthen economic monitoring, and thus to control discretionary decisions more directly. It mandates that the monitor committees must be composed of an equal number of representatives (usually three) from the sickness funds and the AIDs. The chairman, a seventh person who has a tie-breaking vote, is to come from each side in alternate years. This structural change strengthens the position of sickness funds in utilization review, since previously the AIDs held a majority on the review committees in most areas.

The new law also provides for more aggressive controls on prescribing. For the first time, sickness funds and AIDs are required to set ceilings on expenditure growth for prescription drugs. (As with the ceilings on expenditures for physicians' services, ceilings on drug expenditures had been tried on a voluntary contractual basis in some areas before the law went into effect.) If the ceiling for drug expenditures is exceeded, the sickness funds and AIDs must examine the pattern of expenditures to determine the cause of the excess. If they find no outside factor, such as an unexpected epidemic or an unforeseen increase in drug prices, then they must conduct individual reviews of physicians' prescribing behavior and impose fines where appropriate. To help physicians prescribe economically, the Special Commission on Drug Information has been established by executive order with a mandate to publish lists of the costs of therapeutically equivalent drugs.

The passage of the HCCCA demonstrates the potency of the cost control issue as a possible springboard for reform of structural elements of the health care system. Health care cost containment is a classic instance of a policy reform whose benefits are widely dispersed among a large population but whose costs are highly concentrated on an organized group of suppliers.[16] The fact that a major reform, with substantial requirements for limiting health expenditures, could be passed at all is remarkable, given the conventional wisdom of political economy that programs with dispersed benefits and concentrated costs are very difficult to pass.

How can we account for the government's ability to pass the Health Care Cost Containment Act—and most notably, to put a ceiling on growth of expenditures for ambulatory care? Three factors seem particularly important. First, the dramatic escalation of health care costs in the 1970s was a sharp increase in the previous (already steep) trend. The sudden change in the rate of expenditure growth made an already existing problem more visible. Second, the entire public pension system was becoming financially unsound, and since a major financial burden of the pension system is contribution to the sickness funds for health insurance of the elderly, reform of the health system was seen as necessary for the pension program to be able to survive. Thus, the constituency for health care reform was enlarged, and the scope of the medical profession's role in the debate was narrowed. Physicians could legitimately argue about the structure of the health care financing system, but they had no expertise to debate the fiscal solvency of the pension system. (One tactic of the Federal Association of Insurance Doctors was to argue that the government should solve the pension problem with measures applied directly and exclusively to the pension system.)[17]

The third and perhaps most crucial element was public opinion about physicians. Although the medical profession in West Germany has consistently ranked at the top of all occupations in prestige with the general public, sympathy for physicians' economic plight declined dramatically in the 1970s. The level of physicians' incomes began to be publicized in the early 1970s,[18] and popular knowledge about physicians' incomes became more accurate. In surveys conducted in 1973 and 1977, respondents typically underestimated physicians' incomes, but in 1977, their guesses were more accurate. And while only twenty percent of respondents in 1973 thought that physicians' incomes were "too high," this was the opinion of fully sixty percent in 1977.[19]

In the controversy over the health care cost containment proposal, the government benefited from enormous popular support. When asked which side they favored in the cost containment controversy, forty percent of citizens would not choose sides, forty-five percent favored the government, and only fifteen percent sided with physicians.[20] Moreover, there was strong support for the specific cost control measures outlined in the government's proposal. The strongest support was for pegging physicians' incomes to the income of other members of society. Eighty-four percent of all respondents favored this measure, and support did not go below eighty percent in any subgroup—blue-collar workers, white-collar workers, low income people, high income people, Social Democratic supporters, Christian Democratic supporters, or even people who felt dissatisfied with their physicians. A proposal to allow more ambulatory care to be provided by hospital physicians and laboratories was supported by seventy-eight percent of respondents. And a proposal to set upper limits on expenditures for prescription drugs was favored by sixty-seven percent.[21] Nevertheless, the Federal Association of Insurance Doctors claimed that a limit on drug expenditures would create mistrust between patients and their physicians.[22]

Widespread public support for the government proposal seemed to be generated by increased public information about physicians' incomes, but tactics of physicians in resisting the proposal then seemed to create more popular antipathy to the medical profession. In some cities, physicians staged mass shutdowns of their offices in protest. In other areas, they threatened to close their offices. In Baden-Württemberg, office-based physicians threatened to cease writing sick leave certificates, filling out death certificates, and reporting contagious diseases to the public health authorities. Demonstrations were held—in Hannover the physicians hired student demonstrators—and leaders of physician organizations threatened nationwide strikes or office shutdowns.[23]

Popular reaction to these tactics was overwhelmingly negative. When asked about physicians' tactics, ninety-four percent of respondents opposed strikes (including eighty-four percent of those who sided with physicians); ninety percent opposed shutdowns of offices; and seventy percent opposed demonstrations and rallies. Opposition was consistently high among supporters of both political parties. The only tactics supported by a majority of citizens were posters, advertisements, and brochures in waiting rooms.[24]

By the time the Health Care Cost Containment Act came up for debate, the regime had gathered strong public support, and physicians had managed to erode some of their high stock of goodwill by engaging in tactics that most of the public thought were excessive. The fight over the HCCCA was long and arduous. Although the original proposal was issued in February 1977 and scheduled to take effect on July 1, 1977, the final bill was not passed until June 24, 1977, amid much last-minute high drama. Office-based physicians were opposed principally to two major provisions of the bill—the pegging of expenditure growth rates for physicians' services to the growth rate of income of other members of society, and the opening up of ambulatory care to hospital-based physicians. On both provisions, a compromise was struck.

Sickness fund expenditures for physician services are now to be tied to several economic indicators, including the average annual wage and salary increase, but since no specific formula is contained in the legislation, the restraining influence of the average wage and salary indicator may be diluted by the influence of other permissible indicators, such as increases in practice costs. Moreover, the original government bill called for negotiation of expenditure ceilings by federal organizations of sickness funds and insurance doctors. The final bill widens the scope of negotiations to the Concerted Action, but gives either the sickness funds or insurance doctors the right to veto an agreement and enter into private negotiations with the other.

The provision allowing hospital-based physicians to provide ambulatory care for members of sickness funds is very weak. In order for hospital-based physicians in the locality to practice ambulatory medicine, a committee composed of five representives of sickness funds and five insurance doctors must certify that the locality has insufficient office-based care, and the hospital director or chief of staff must certify that hospital care will not suffer if a physician spends some time in ambulatory practice.

The strongest defeat for the government came on its proposal for cost containment in the hospital sector. The government had wanted to impose some controls on the hospital sector, and these provisions in the Ministry of Labor's original bill are notably absent in the final product. Missing are the provisions which would have required hospitals to bear ten percent of the cost of all new building projects and five percent of the cost of renovations, and which would have established that the per diem rates be negotiated between statewide organizations of sickness funds and hospitals, instead of the current system of rate-setting by state agencies with advice of the sickness funds. Since hospital services are the fastest growing sector of health expenditures, the defeat on these provisions was a significant setback.

The HCCCA mandated a comprehensive restructuring of the German health insurance system. Yet, like most revolutions, it came about at a time when things were getting better, not worse. Annual growth rates of expenditures for all types of health services had begun to slow down in 1975, and showed a substantial decrease in 1976 (see table 9.2).

In its first year, the reform seemed to be a huge success. The annual increase in health expenditures under the public health insurance program slowed to about 7 percent, and for the first time in many years, the annual increase in expenditures by the local sickness funds was lower than the increase in the nation's average wage and salary. The National Health Commission was able to reach an agreement to limit expenditures for physicians' services in fiscal 1979 to an increase of 5.5 percent over the 1978 level.

Unfortunately, the damping effect of the new law has been short-lived. Preliminary figures for 1979 indicate that rates of growth for the major categories of expenditure are back up to their pre-1976 levels. Analysts have begun to realize that the reduced expenditure growth rates in the mid-1970s were the result of a combination of special factors. Most important among these was the "shock effect" of a sudden anti-physician sentiment in a broad-based political coalition and in public opinion. Much of the initial slowdown was attributable to physicians' voluntary restraint in the face of more severe measures.

The compromises of the Health Care Cost Containment Act reflect the changing balance of power in the health sector. Office-based physicians are no longer able to win all their conflicts through collective action, as they did in the early part of the century, and the government has been able to win a significant political victory. Whether the HCCCA itself will actually restrain costs in the long run is a question that is open to much speculation. But the important symbolic victory for the government and the sickness funds is incontrovertible—there is clearly strong popular support for imposing limits on the collective and discretionary power of office-based physicians. The enormous political strength of the hospital sector, reflected in its ability to defeat almost every provision of the bill affecting hospitals, underlines the increasing importance of the *Länder* and the hospitals as the locus for new technology, the employer of the majority of physicians and health professionals, and the object of a major portion of public expenditures.

Chapter Ten | Conclusion: Lessons for the United States

The political integration of technical experts is a problem facing all modern societies. Philosophers and social scientists have argued that knowledge, rather than property, is becoming the mark of a new elite.[1] The problem facing modern political systems is to develop mechanisms for controlling power based on knowledge and for rendering the new technical elite more accountable to the rest of society.

The medical profession represents one very important example of this problem. Physicians provide a kind of technical expertise that is highly valued, and physicians are among economic and social elites in all Western countries. As health and illness come to be understood as phenomena amenable to human intervention, and as governments assume more responsibility for citizen health and health care, physicians become increasingly important as political advisers to government, as providers of a valued service, and as allocators of government benefits.

The medical profession has its own unique characteristics that distinguish its practitioners from other types of technical experts. It is a relatively old profession, even though some of its technology and much of its ability to influence the course of disease is very new. Medical care touches on the personal lives of most people with an impact that few, if any, other kinds of technical expertise can be said to have. And the medical profession operates in the context of deeply embedded cultural notions about the nature of disease, of science, and of medical care, which are not often a part of the ideological framework of other kinds of technical experts. Nevertheless, an understanding of the ways that societies have attempted to integrate their medical professions may be instructive not only for the problem of physicians' power, but also for the more general problem of how technical expertise can be optimally utilized but still made responsive to agendas set in a democratic context.

The collective power of West German physicians is institutionalized in several ways that also partially neutralize that power. The medical profession was integrated politically into the state in a manner that was analogous to other occupational groups. The profession was not defined as a group that required special treatment with respect to the degree of control by government, but rather was established as a self-regulating corporative occupational chamber following the preexisting pattern for other occupations.

The rationales that support self-regulation by the medical profession are quite different in Germany and the United States. In both countries, the inherent technical complexity of medical science and the technical expertise of physicians are important arguments that favor professional independence from government regulation. But the political arguments that support the right of the medical profession to govern itself are very different and lead to different degrees of professional independence from state control.

In Germany, self-regulation is grounded in a conception of society as an organic whole whose constituent parts are large social groups based primarily on economic functions. The interests of individuals are best guaranteed through their membership in the appropriate social groups, which in turn regulate the behavior of individual members in accordance with the group's collective purpose. The state then serves as a coordinator of all the corporative groups, making sure that all subscribe to some basic ground rules and the behavior of each is consistent with the national interest. Thus, the corporatist view of politics in Germany has provided strong justification for government oversight of medical affairs.

The delegation of governmental authority to the American medical profession is by no means an anomaly within the context of American politics. Grant McConnell has demonstrated that American democratic theory rests on a strong tradition of fostering government by private associations.[2] Not only is power delegated from one branch of the government to another, but government allows private groups to control certain areas of policy autonomously. Business corporations and unions are two notable examples of private associations which are allowed to determine rules that govern behavior of individuals and groups within some limited sphere of policy.

The ideological justifications for allowing private associations to govern themselves (and their members) are based on the special character of private associations. Certain traits of private associations are thought to justify departure from a requirement of democratic internal organization and from serious supervision by, or responsibility to, democratic institutions of the state.[3] First, private associations are thought to involve voluntary participation of their members, in contrast to a town, state, or nation, whose citizens have very little choice about whether or not to be citizens; hence, the potential for coercion is thought to be low. Second, private associations are meetings of like-minded people who share some common interest; given the homogeneity of the membership, there is unlikely to be very much internal conflict that would need to be resolved through democratic structures of government.

And finally, private associations have a limited purpose. They will limit their activities to matters concerned with their specific purpose, and therefore there is no cause for concern that they might become too powerful and encroach on other areas of their members' lives. The medical profession in the United States has benefited from all of these arguments for independence from government control. In addition, the arguments of technical expertise and of the therapeutic value of a personal doctor-patient relationship support a policy of noninterference by the government.

The different ideological grounds for professional freedom from government control in West Germany and the United States lead to rather different policy implications. In the United States, the medical profession and other private associations have been granted political autonomy largely because their affairs are not thought to be of great political significance either to their individual members or to the state as a whole. In Germany, the medical profession has been allowed to regulate itself because the dominant ideology holds that all important social and economic functions are best performed by self-regulating corporative groups. Thus, in the United States the basic question in the relationship between physicians and government is whether there should be any government control over medical affairs at all. In Germany, the question has always been what kind of government regulation is appropriate for the medical profession.

The German medical profession seems to derive its collective power primarily from its early willingness to engage in collective action against both the state and private employers. Because German physicians were heavily dependent on employment by sickness funds from very early on, the image of the independent, self-employed, free practitioner was not so firmly embedded in the profession's collective self image as it has been for the American medical profession. The German medical profession formed a strong trade union organization whose explicit purpose was to improve job security and professional freedom in the practice of medicine. Members of the Leipziger Verband engaged in strikes, boycotts, and other collective actions designed to accomplish these purposes. The organization's success in attracting physician members indicates that the majority of physicians did not see any conflict or inconsistency between the image of a "professional" and that of a "worker."

The willingness of German physicians to organize themselves as a trade union contrasts sharply with the history of the American medical profession. Undoubtedly this difference in mentality can be largely explained by the difference between the employment conditions of the two professions. The American profession has been, and continues to be, dominated by a large majority of office-based self-employed physicians. The unionization of physicians has only recently begun in the United States, and then mostly among house staff physicians who are salaried employees of hospitals.[4] The issue of legitimacy of physician unions and strikes is far from settled among the profession, as any perusal of letters to trade journals or surveys of physicians' attitudes will show. American physicians' increasing acceptance of unionization as a political strategy is one way that the American and German health care systems seem to be converging. If the German experience gives us any indication, then as the structure of the American profession shifts toward salaried employment, or even a high dependence on government payment programs, American physicians will have a greater propensity to form unions and use union tactics to protect their interests.

Beyond the trade union organization of physicians, certain government decisions explicitly strengthened physicians' associations in health policy in West Germany. Aside from the indirect effect of public health insurance as a stimulus to trade union organization among physicians, government decisions in the early 1930s created the associations of insurance doctors as monopolistic organizations. The AIDs were created by government fiat and then fell under the control of the only really powerful physicians' organization, the Hartmanbund, whose own political purpose was to protect the jobs and autonomy of practice of its physician members. In the second year after their formation, the AIDs were then given exclusive rights to negotiate with sickness funds to provide medical care to fund members, and collective contracts replaced all individual contracting.

Government decisions have also enhanced the political authority of West German physicians as individuals. Any public program which distributes benefits contingent on medical illness necessarily puts physicians in the position of allocating benefits. Under West Germany's national health insurance, physicians are the key decisionmakers about the nature and volume of medical goods and services purchased by the members of the social insurance program. Of course, it is true that physicians are always highly influential, if not determinative, in the selection of medical goods and services, even when the source of payment is totally private. But the very existence of a public program for financing health services in a sense magnifies the discretionary power of physicians so that they are making decisions about public resources as well as private.

In the United States, the introduction of some public financing of medical care through Medicare and Medicaid has had precisely this effect of politicizing what were once purely medical decisions. Through public insurance, physicians have taken on an additional role as spending agents for the government. In response to the realization that physicians are indeed controlling a significant share of social resources, Americans have introduced several programs designed to render physicians more accountable to some conception of the public interest. Exactly what "the public interest" is with respect to medical care is a matter of vigorous public debate, but the purpose of many new government programs is essentially the same: to put some kind of restraint on the power of physicians to allocate public resources. Two such programs bear striking similarities to mechanisms West Germany has used: professional standards review organizations and health maintenance organizations.

Lessons about Utilization Review

Professional standards review organizations (PSROs) are peer review organizations mandated by Congress in the Social Security amendments of 1972.[5] The program is a response to the failure of previously existing mechanisms to control adequately the costs of the Medicare and Medicaid programs. Those mechanisms—utilization review committees for hospital services, and claims review by Medicare intermediaries—were considered too fragmented, inconsistently applied, poorly accepted by physicians, and largely ineffective.[6] The PSRO program is designed to impose some cost and quality controls on medical services that are paid for by the Social Security Administration (primarily Medicare and Medicaid benefits). The original PSRO legislation called for review of care provided in institutional settings, such as hospitals and nursing homes. Review of outpatient and office care is expected to be performed by PSROs within two years of designation as a PSRO.

The legislation calls for the Department of Health, Education, and Welfare (HEW) to designate "qualified organizations" as PSROs to perform a review of medical care in their respective jurisdictions. A qualified organization is, according to the law, a nonprofit professional association composed of licensed physicians and osteopaths, whose membership is voluntary, open to all physicians and osteopaths in the area, and includes a "substantial portion" of them. A PSRO may not require that its members either belong to or pay dues to any organized medical society or association.[7] This definitely eliminates medical societies and in effect limits eligibility to foundations for medical care. These are business associations of physicians established to provide health services and/or claims review; often they are sponsored and organized by medical societies, though they are themselves autonomous corporations.[8]

The development of PSROs is analogous to the development of AIDs in that both were suddenly called into existence by federal legislation or decree. In the resulting power vacuum, established professional political organizations were easily able to dominate the new organizations. In the American case, several previously existing foundations for medical care were the first organizations to receive conditional PSRO contracts.[9] In regions where there are no existing foundations or other qualified organizations, state and county medical societies are in the best position to organize PSROs, simply because they have the organizational capital and because the PSROs must be composed of physicians.

The purpose of PSRO review is to determine whether federally financed medical services are "medically necessary"; of a quality consistent with "professionally recognized standards of health care"; and provided in the most economical and effective kind of health care facility.[10] These general criteria for review are meant to stimulate both cost and quality control. Cost control is implicit in the first and third criteria; peer review is intended to cut down on the sheer volume of services rendered (and thus on the absolute total of health care costs) by eliminating "medically unnecessary" services, and to discourage the use of expensive facilities when less expensive ones could provide equally effective service.[11] Quality control is implicit in the first two general criteria— "medical necessity" and "professionally recognized standards of health care." In order to carry out quality control, PSROs are mandated to establish "norms of care, diagnosis, and treatment based upon typical patterns of practice" in the PSRO area.[12] These norms might include indications for a given therapy; volume of treatment (e.g., length of stay in a hospital, drug dosages) for a given diagnosis; and adequacy of care (recommended services for a given diagnosis). PSROs are also directed to establish and maintain "profiles of care" for patients and "providers" (doctors and hospitals). Presumably these profiles will be used as a screening device to single out extraordinary cases and patterns of practice for closer review.

In order to conduct their review, PSROs are given the authority to examine the records of doctors and institutions and to inspect the facilities where publicly financed care is provided. PSROs have two sanctions available to help ensure compliance of doctors and hospitals. Upon recommendation of a PSRO, the secretary of HEW may deny a doctor or hospital eligibility to participate in Medicare and Medicaid (i.e., to be reimbursed by the government for services provided). Alternatively, the secretary may impose a fee on the offending doctor or hospital as a condition for continued eligibility; the fee is to be equal to the cost of the services that were deemed medically unnecessary or improper, or $5,000, whichever is less.

The American system of professional standards review differs from West German economic monitoring in several important ways. The German utilization review applies only to services provided in an office by an office doctor, while the PSROs may review only institutional care. Although both programs provide for review of publicly financed care only, the public sector in Germany accounts for a much greater proportion of total health services costs. Another major difference is that the PSROs are supposed to develop explicit norms for quality of care. Economic monitoring uses only one formal norm for the first stage of screening—the average cost (or claim) per patient. Quality indicators are applied only informally in the subjective decisions of monitor doctors, though they may use profiles of care developed for the AIDs as their guidelines. Finally, in the West German system there is an organized adversary to the associations of insurance doctors—the sickness funds. Sickness funds have the right to challenge decisions of the monitor committees and to have their own doctors participate in the grievance committees which decide appeals, and as of 1977, sickness funds are entitled to parity representation on monitor committees.

Despite these differences, professional standards review is strikingly similar to economic monitoring. Both programs impose compulsory review of services financed through the public sector. In both systems, the review is performed by organizations of physicians that receive their mandate and authority directly from the federal government. In both, the review organizations develop physician and patient profiles using regional norms of practice. Review is on a case-by-case basis. Both systems use "process standards"; that is, they evaluate the services and procedures provided for the patient, rather than the facilities provided ("input standards") or the results of care ("outcome standards"). In both systems, the sanctions against doctors are denial of reimbursement for particular procedures, and in extraordinary cases, denial of eligibility to participate in the insurance program. Finally, in both programs, the initiative for discipline is in the hands of the physicians' organizations.

The West German experience with government mandated peer review of physicians' services should lead us to be very skeptical about the ability of PSROs to constrain public health expenditures. After 1968, as the system of prospectively negotiated fixed pools was abandoned and economic monitoring became virtually the only bulwark against rapid expenditure growth, expenditures for physicians' services grew at an average annual rate of over fifteen percent, as compared with about ten percent per year in the preceding decade.[13] While expenditure growth might conceivably have been greater had there been no utilization review, most analysts would agree that a fifteen percent annual growth rate is unacceptably high. Thus, without expenditure ceilings, utilization review as practiced in West Germany was unable to provide enough control on physicians' services.

This failure of utilization review as a cost control mechanism in West Germany is especially significant for Americans, because economic monitoring has several features that should make it more rather than less likely to succeed than PSROs. First, the original legislative standards for economic monitoring provided a stronger basis for limiting care than the legislative standards for PSROs. The RVO specified that care must be "sufficient and appropriate, but may not exceed that which is necessary." The original health insurance program was clearly meant to provide some minimum level of coverage. The RVO contained the implication that, for any given disease, there is some level of care that is necessary and sufficient to achieve a cure, and national health insurance provided an entitlement to precisely that level of care. There was no explicit entitlement to high quality services. But even such strong legislative criteria have proved nearly useless as a means of setting clear limits on what society will pay for. Under pressure of constant legal challenges, the courts have resorted to professional definitions of "sufficient and necessary" to resolve controversies in specific instances.

The American PSRO legislation, by contrast, contains language that makes quality assurance and cost control both objectives of the program right from the beginning. This legislative ambiguity about the purpose of PSROs led to an immediate struggle during the implementation of the program between advocates of a tough, cost-cutting program and advocates of professional freedom to determine the services for which public health insurance would pay. "In the rhetoric of this highly politicized debate, 'quality of care' became something of a 'code word' for professional prerogatives, and 'cost control' was soft-pedaled, having become a 'buzz word' for government interference."[14] Responsibility for implementation and oversight of PSROs, instead of being given to the Social Security Administration, which administered the payments for Medicare and Medicaid and which had a stake in fiscal control, was lodged in the Office of the Assistant Secretary for Health, which has traditionally been concerned with promoting health services development and has been very responsive to the interests of organized medicine. The newly created Office of Professional Standards Review, in order to gain the cooperation of physicians that it felt was essential for program success, publicly proclaimed that quality assurance was the primary goal of PSROs.[15] Thus, whereas the West German economic monitoring system was established and operated for many years under a mandate to determine minimally necessary levels of care, American PSROs from the very beginning have been organized to assure high quality services.

A second feature of economic monitoring that should make it stronger than the PSRO system is the representation of third-party payors on the review committees. PSROs are composed entirely of physicians, but economic monitoring committees have had representatives of the sickness funds since the transition to a fee-for-service method of calculating the pool. Until 1977, sickness funds were rarely given majority (or even parity) on the committees, so there is no way of knowing whether economic monitoring might be more effective if third-party payors were granted more authority. But if utilization review with *some* participation by third-party payors is unable to provide much restraint in West Germany, it is unlikely that utilization review with *no* consumer or payor representation will be any stronger in the United States.

Finally, economic monitoring is a system that has had the benefits of time and experience. It had been in place for nearly forty years when it was confronted with the task of controlling physicians' services without a fixed pool to act as a brake. The AIDs have a large network of accounting offices and comprehensive data collection and processing systems. If professionally controlled utilization review could be expected to work anywhere, it should have worked in West Germany. The very fact that West German policymakers found it necessary to reassert expenditure ceilings in 1977 should deter American policymakers from relying on utilization review as the primary cost control device in any national health insurance program.

The West German experience with government mandated peer review should also lead us to appreciate the tendency of bureaucratic regulation to influence the orientation of practice toward the accounting norms used in the system. Economic monitoring, like PSROs, uses process norms, and critics of the system have argued that it creates a technical bias in the practice of medicine.[16] Because doctors can be reimbursed only for procedures coded in the fee schedule, the economic incentive is to perform procedures, rather than to spend a long time taking a history, explaining, advising, or reassuring. Moreover, the relatively low fees allowed for consultations and examinations are additional disincentives for doctors to spend time talking with patients.

Even without the influence of bureaucratic regulation, American medicine has been shaped by what Victor Fuchs has aptly called a "technologic imperative." In Fuchs's words, "Medical tradition emphasizes giving the best care that is technologically possible; the only legitimate and explicitly recognized constraint is the state of the art."[17] A technical bias in medicine may be as much the result of medical education and training as of fee schedules and fee-for-service reimbursement. But at least one study of different methods of peer review suggests that the very method by which physicians evaluate each other may contribute significantly to their technical bias. It was found that when physicians use explicit process norms (i.e., formal lists of procedures that constitute "good care" for specific diagnoses), they are likely to expect many more procedures to be performed than normally are.[18] Only two percent of the cases evaluated were found to provide an acceptable level of care when judged by explicit process norms. The same cases, when judged by outcome criteria or by subjective process criteria, were evaluated much more highly, with as many as sixty-three percent being found "adequate." This study suggests that the use of process criteria in evaluating the quality of care leads physicians to use an academic standard ("Was everything possible done for this patient?") rather than an economic standard of care. Thus, although PSROs are supposed to evaluate the "medical necessity" of treatment, the development of explicit criteria of care may lead them to apply a very broad definition of medical necessity. The use of process criteria by PSROs may only exacerbate the technical and interventionist bias of current medical practice, a development that certainly will not curb the cost of medical care.

West Germany's experience is also illustrative of how reimbursement of physicians according to fee schedules shapes the practice of medicine by setting the relative prices of various sectors of medical practice. The reliance on a fee schedule means that the relative fees for various kinds of medical procedures at one point in time become frozen and serve to set the prices for some unspecified period in the future. This is true not only because there is a practical limit to the frequency with which new schedules can be set, but also because strong political interests develop around the higher priced sectors of medical care. The setting of prices also serves as an incentive for all doctors to invest in equipment in the higher priced sectors, especially when any type of doctor can be reimbursed for procedures in any specialty. Once the investment is made a substantial part of the profession has a stake in preserving the status quo of the fee schedule. The reimbursement system based on periodically renegotiated fee schedules seems to cause some technological lags, in the sense that there may be an economic incentive for older technologies to continue to be used even when their medical value has declined relative to other methods of care.

The technological rigidities caused by the reimbursement mechanisms in West Germany may arise because economic monitoring relies almost exclusively on cost norms. The fact that PSROs will use norms based purely on medical process (e.g., criteria for hospital admission, criteria for discharge, length-of-stay norms for specific diseases) rather than cost norms does not mean that the West German experience is irrelevant to our own. It suggests that broad organizational interests may develop around any kind of norm, and that when norms reflect the balance of power or the majority mode of practice (as norms are likely to do), they may be very difficult to change.[19]

Finally, the cost of administering the economic monitoring system itself should give us pause about the possibilities of PSROs as a cost saving device. In chapter 7 it was noted that the administrative costs of the AIDs are approximately ten times greater than the money saved through cutbacks of doctors' reimbursements. Even allowing for the likelihood that some proportion of the AIDs' administrative costs may be used for purposes other than running the monitoring system, these figures suggest that a highly bureaucratic peer review system is likely to generate substantial costs of its own.

Lessons for Health Maintenance Organizations

Another major movement in American health policy reform has been the promotion and development of health maintenance organizations (HMOs). HMOs are comprehensive financing and service plans for the provision of medical care to a group of subscribers. There are many varieties of HMOs (and many names), but essentially all share three basic characteristics: they finance themselves through prepaid contributions from their members, and therefore have a fixed budget; they offer a fixed, stated range of services, all of which are covered by the prepayment; and they have a fixed population of enrollees. The basic differences among HMOs have to do with the degree of control each exerts over the providers of care to its subscribers. Some, like Kaiser Permanente and Group Health Cooperative of Puget Sound, operate their own outpatient clinics and hospitals. Others, such as Health Insurance Plan of New York, have their own outpatient clinics but contract with area hospitals for inpatient care. The least degree of control is represented by HMOs which contract with individual physicians and area hospitals and reimburse on a fee-for-service basis. This model describes many of the medical care foundations, such as San Joaquin Medical Foundation in California. The basic feature of all three types is that they operate with a fixed budget and therefore presumably have a strong incentive to be cost conscious.

HMOs have been touted by their proponents as a vehicle for restructuring the American health care system and as a potential device for lowering health care costs, improving access to services, and increasing the quality of medical care.[20] Health maintenance organizations are not entirely new in the United States, although they have not always been graced with the title. The Kaiser Permanente Health Plan was started for Kaiser employees in 1946, and since then Group Health Cooperative of Puget Sound, the Health Insurance Plan of New York, and many other comprehensive prepaid health plans have come into existence. Although such organizations have been around for a long time and have had small groups of advocates here and there, it has been relatively recently that government has looked to HMOs as a strategy for solving national health policy problems. The idea of using HMOs as a cost saving device was picked up by the Nixon Administration in 1970, and by the end of 1973 a health maintenance organization act had been passed by Congress.[21] The act provides for federal funding to stimulate the formation of HMOs but also specifies a fairly stringent set of requirements which applicants must meet in order to be eligible for the funds. Development of HMOs has been much slower than supporters had hoped; in 1972 Secretary of HEW Elliot Richardson predicted the establishment of sixteen hundred HMOs by 1980, but more current estimates foresee only about seventy or eighty HMOs by that time.[22]

Meanwhile, there have been numerous studies attempting to evaluate the potential of HMOs to fulfill their promises,[23] and since the evidence is still inconclusive, it would be worthwhile to add to these studies some evidence from health systems abroad. The West German system of health insurance through sickness funds certainly has many of the elements of the health maintenance organization strategy, and the present case study suggests that there are a few lessons to be learned.

Like HMOs, sickness funds provide health services for a defined population of members. Members pay a fixed contribution, and until the late 1960s, most funds operated on a relatively fixed budget. The range of services they must provide is specified by law, and these services together with the optional benefits offered by each fund make up a fixed package of benefits. Sickness funds are most like the foundation model of an HMO described above, where the HMO contracts with individual physicians to provide services. Although sickness funds now use collective contracts with AIDs rather than individual contracts, physicians are ultimately reimbursed on a fee-for-service basis, and even the pool is established with reference to fee-for-service claims. Despite the differences in some of the organizational details, the system of health insurance in West Germany originally embodied the core principle of the HMO strategy: fixed budgeting by numerous membership groups.

One clear lesson from West Germany is that political support for fixed budget health plans is very unstable when these plans coexist with plans that reimburse on an open-ended, fee-for-service basis. When HMOs are forced to compete with health insurance plans that control costs less aggressively, the HMOs may be very vulnerable to charges of providing second-class care. In the West German situation, both the medical definition of "necessary and appropriate" services, and the popular definition that derives from the medical definition, are set by physicians treating privately insured patients. Few, if any, social institutions can withstand the pressure to "keep up" with high-status, private-sector medicine. The substitute sickness funds feel compelled to offer the same services as the private health insurance plans, and the RVO funds are then under pressure to match the substitute funds. The legislature seems unwilling to set firm ceilings on the funds' tax rates, and instead allows expanded benefits to be financed by a regressive taxing scheme. The courts, when confronted with the task of defining the scope of services to be provided under national health insurance, retreat to an acceptance of professional standards.

Another obvious lesson from West Germany is that expenditure controls that do not apply to the entire health care market may not be very effective if there is significant use of health services outside the publicly controlled system. It is sobering to note that expenditures outside the social insurance system in Germany remain quite important, despite the long historical tradition of sickness funds and their generally high acceptability to the West German people. The absence of a tradition of consumer membership societies for the provision of health services in the United States means that the non-HMO sector is likely to be even more tenacious.

Given the rather slow rate of development of HMOs in the United States, their effect on health care expenditures is apt to be rather minimal. Less than five percent of Americans belong to HMOs,[24] and numerous studies have revealed that members often use out-of-plan services, despite the strong economic incentive to use only HMO-provided services. Estimates of out-of-plan use by members of the Kaiser Permanente plan are diverse: 10 percent of all subscribers in one study;[25] 12 percent of all subscribers for office care and 7.2 percent of subscribers for hospital care in another study;[26] 44 percent of subscribers in still another study;[27] and as many as 55 percent of subscribers in a consumer satisfaction survey.[28] However one reconciles these estimates, it is clear that out-of-plan use is not insignificant. Each HMO may itself operate on a fixed budget, and thus have a strong incentive to curb the "do-everything" mentality of its panel physicians, but if there is a steady "leakage" of patients into the non-HMO sector (and if the HMO sector is extremely small to begin with), it is unlikely that HMOs will be very effective in controlling health care expenditures.

The proponents of HMOs think that these plans will be likely to alter traditional patterns of practice, particularly with respect to the balance between preventive and curative care. Because HMOs cover ambulatory care (unlike most Blue Cross/Blue Shield and private insurance plans), and because they have a limited budget, HMOs are alleged to provide more preventive screening and early treatment and thus avoid more expensive care for advanced diseases. Empirical evidence on this question is mixed, and in any case there is certainly no strong evidence in support of the argument.[29]

The evidence from West Germany is also quite mixed. Through the sickness funds the government has been able to institute a nationwide program of preventive screening examinations for children and adults. Nevertheless, one would have to conclude that there is little evidence that the West German system has been able to reorient patterns of medical care away from technical procedures and toward a concept of social medicine that emphasizes patient education, counseling, and preventive care, even with a much more highly developed HMO-like system than the United States is likely to have in the foreseeable future.

Lessons for Nonmedical Benefit Programs

Another area where the West German system offers some fruitful lessons to the United States is in the use of physicians as gatekeepers for nonmedical benefits and privileges. The German system of wage continuation payments based on sick leave certificates is probably more significant in monetary terms than any single illness-related nonmedical benefit program in the United States. Nevertheless, there are numerous activities and benefits in the United States which are somehow contingent on certification of illness (or sometimes health) by a physician. Cash benefits under workmen's compensation programs, veterans' disability pensions, Social Security disability insurance, and other disability insurance programs are contingent on certification of injury by a physician. Exemption from military service (until the end of the draft), jury duty, and testifying in court can all be obtained by some kind of certification of illness. Mental illness, as certified by a psychiatrist, may provide an exemption from the normal sanctions against criminal violations. Under some circumstances, a certification of mental or physical illness may entitle a woman to obtain a legal abortion which would otherwise be illegal. Some state welfare programs include extra grants for recipients who obtain a physician's certification of medical necessity for a special diet. And finally, insurance companies usually require a physical examination and statement of health by a physician before they will issue a life insurance policy.

Perhaps the most important observation about the West German system of illness certification is that transferring authority to physicians for what is essentially a redistributive program does not depoliticize the redistributive issues. Employer and employee unions, as well as sickness funds, continue to engage in heated polemics about whether the workers are receiving "too much" money through the program. The debate is couched in terms of whether there is "malingering" and whether doctors are too "lenient" in writing certificates, but the central issue is clearly income redistribution. Although the system of wage continuation payments has existed in some scope and form since before the national health insurance program, the program continues to be a major political issue and as recently as 1969 led to a major social policy initiative by the Social Democratic government.

Even where allocation of some nonmedical benefits is based on a formalized system of medical examination and certification, the distribution of benefits may still be class related. Despite the cultural paradigm of medicine as "objective" and "neutral" with respect to social and political divisions, the evidence presented in chapter 8 indicates that a program based ostensibly on medical decisions can in fact disguise serious differences in the treatment of different social groups. Class differences are evident at both stages of the process. The rate of summonses to the board of control doctors is twice as high for blue-collar workers (10 percent of all certificates) as for white-collar workers (5 percent of all certificates). And once patients reach the board, they are more likely to be found eligible for continued payments if they are high-income, white-collar workers than if they are lower income (compulsorily insured), blue-collar workers.

Future research in the United States could profitably examine the nature and effect of distributive systems that use physicians as gatekeepers. One study of draft exemptions during the 1960s found that the rate of medical disqualifications for whites was about ten percent higher than for blacks.[30] Similar studies are needed for other kinds of benefit programs that are distributed ostensibly on the basis of medical criteria. Some monitoring of these programs, either by physicians or other experts (perhaps even statisticians), may be necessary to help ensure that the benefits are in fact distributed according to reasonable criteria of need.

Lessons for National Health Insurance

Advocates of national health insurance in the United States have usually been divided into two camps. On one side are supporters of a plan that would provide universal coverage (i.e., all citizens would be covered) and comprehensive benefits (i.e., most types of medical services would be covered, including outpatient care, preventive services, hospital care, and services for the critically ill, the chronically ill, and the disabled). On the other side are supporters of plans that would limit coverage to some subgroup of the population, and/or limit benefits to some particular types of services. In the 1970s, when health care cost control became a major political concern, national health insurance plans of the limited variety gained increasing favor. The West German national health insurance system, though now nearly universal and comprehensive, has evolved through various stages of development in which coverage applied only to limited groups and limited types of services. The German system thus offers some lessons about the consequences of different types of designs.

The most important lesson from West Germany is that once any kind of national health insurance program is begun, it will expand, both in number of people covered and types of services or benefits provided. The West German system was introduced and designed by a Conservative government wishing to provide *minimum* income protection to a small, clearly defined group of citizens. Both the statutory language defining the program and the organizational devices used to administer it were designed to place clear limits on the population served and benefits provided. Nevertheless, once even a minimal national health insurance system was in place, so was the potential for expansion by more liberal or socialist governments.

No matter what small group of "needy" people is identified as requiring government health insurance, there will be continual pressures to include other groups, until nearly the whole population is covered. Already the Medicaid and Medicare programs have generated pressures to expand government health insurance. Particularly where an income level is used to define the eligibility for a program (as in Medicaid), there will always be some group with incomes just above the limit for whom the expenses associated with illness will be a significant burden.

Similarly, no matter how carefully a legislature tries to define the services covered by a limited national health insurance program, there will be continual pressure to broaden the scope of benefits. The method of limiting benefits that seems to be politically most attractive in the United States is to create national health insurance for "catastrophic" expenses only. "Catastrophic" might be defined as expenses above some monetary amount, or as expenses associated with particular diseases known to require expensive treatment, such as kidney disease. Either definition is inherently expansive. Medical research and new technology will create more and more ways of treating people that are "catastrophically" expensive, and policymakers will find it difficult to resist the argument that social justice requires doing everything within the scope of medical science.

Another conception of national health insurance that has had serious support from the Nixon, Ford, and Carter administrations is a program that would offer different benefit packages to different social groups. Thus, for example, employed persons would be in one plan, low-income and unemployed in another, the aged in still another.[31] The plans would be financed slightly differently and would offer different benefit levels to their members. Another less restrictive version would *finance* health services differently for the aged, the poor, and others (using vouchers and tax credits), but would allow each person to apply his federal subsidy to the cost of any qualified health plan.[32] The West German national health insurance system is precisely such a system—a conglomeration of separate plans for different social groups, each offering different benefits, but all regulated by some minimal criteria established at the federal level.

The argument for a multitiered system is that marketlike incentives for efficiency will be created if consumers are allowed to choose among different benefit packages with different price tags, and if consumers have to pay at least some of the costs of any package.[33] Arguments for a multitiered system based on market analogies assume that competition in the health system will be driven by suppliers who offer "efficient," low-cost services. In fact, the system will more likely be driven by the suppliers who offer the highest cost services. This is because neither consumers, nor physicians, nor policymakers have any way of comparing outcomes of different services, so they all rely on the implicit guideline that "more is better."

The West German system illustrates that the different health insurance plans (in this case sickness funds) do not compete for voluntary members on the basis of lower costs, but rather, higher quality. Since there are no outcome measures of health service quality, high expenditures are taken by both fund administrators and consumer/citizens as a proxy for quality. High expenditures by sickness funds become a virtue, a mark of high quality, and a symbol of social status. The standards for the whole system are set by the level of services provided by the health insurance for the rich. If the rich choose to pay higher premiums, get broader coverage, and pay for a lot of amenities through their health insurance premiums, they will create similar demands among people covered in other health insurance plans. The West German experience shows that when a government sponsors different "levels" of health insurance plans, it faces a choice of allowing the high expenditure, high status plans to set the general standard, or of incurring the anger and hostility of low expenditure, low status plan members.

This dynamic means that government cannot rely on consumer choice among multiple plans to keep health expenditures down. Some outside standards must be set. There are several ways that standards could be imposed on the health insurance system. One is to create one standard benefit package for everyone, and either eliminate or minimize private health insurance. Since no non-socialist country has eliminated private health insurance, this is not really an option. But policymakers should be aware that if substantial private insurance is allowed to coexist with public insurance, private plans will be forced to offer "better coverage" to their members in order to woo customers away from the public coverage, and the private insurance plans will then set the political standard for the public insurance plans.

Another method of setting standards is to allow physicians to define the services that are necessary and sufficient to treat each particular type of medical problem. The drawback of this method is that physicians are motivated to define the standards in a way that gives them the most possible freedom in therapeutic choices. By themselves, they have no incentives to set standards narrowly. And even when third-party payors are given some role in applying the standards, utilization review by itself does not seem to be a strong constraining device.

A third option is for government to avoid setting standards (either itself, or through physicians' organizations), but simply to set expenditure ceilings. Expenditure ceilings might be set by limits on revenue raising capacity of health insurance bodies, by direct government limits on expenditures, or by voluntary agreements. When agreements between payors and providers are the mechanism for setting ceilings, the success of the mechanism will depend on the strength of payors as a countervailing power. Where physicians are confronted by a multitude of different health insurance plans, any differences in expenditures by the different plans will generate pressures for the "poorer" or lower paying plans to keep up with the more expensive higher paying plans.

Lessons about the Political Integration of Physicians

The West German health insurance system represents another theory about how a society can control the power of its technical experts. In that theory, the power of an expert group is consolidated by deliberate legal arrangements, but then confronted by a countervailing power that is also the creation of political arrangements. In practice, the West German health insurance system is not the "best case" on which to test the efficacy of the theory. The sickness funds have been considerably weakened by the internal competition among themselves. If the countervailing power strategy is to work, government needs to take steps to assure that both sides have approximately equal strength.

Despite the weakness of sickness funds as organized adversaries, they have managed to achieve some successes. The RVO funds were able to negotiate a nationwide agreement on expenditure ceilings for physicians' services. More importantly, they formed the core of support for the efforts of the executive branch to restructure the health insurance system in pursuit of cost control objectives. The government's effort was not entirely successful—but significant legislation was passed, and health expenditure growth has been considerably slowed. Whether the reductions are the result of fear that regulation would be even worse than voluntary restraint, or whether the reductions are the direct result of government regulation, West Germany has achieved dramatic reductions in its health expenditure growth. It might well be that the most effective government tool for getting professions to regulate themselves responsibly is to generate fear that government regulation is terrible and imminent.

Policymakers, as well as academic observers, tend to accept certain assumptions about the behavior of actors and institutions in the health care sector, either because these assumptions are part of our shared intellectual heritage or because they "seem logical" and there is no evidence to disprove them. The experiences of other countries may well provide empirical evidence on some of these questions and may also challenge us to consider solutions that would not be generated within our own intellectual paradigms. But the most important value of comparative case studies is that they emphasize that the political power of the medical profession is an artifact of political arrangements as well as technical expertise. And once policymakers appreciate that lesson, they should be optimistic about the potential for reform.

1. Two excellent works that examine specific uses of power by the American Medical Association are: "The American Medical Association: Power, Purpose and Politics in Organized Medicine," *Yale Law Journal* 63 (May 1954): 938–1029; and Elton Rayack, *Professional Power and American Medicine* (Cleveland: World, 1967).

2. Eliot Freidson, *Profession of Medicine* (New York: Dodd, Mead, 1970).

3. Ibid., pp. 45–55.

4. Odin Anderson, *Uneasy Equilibrium* (New Haven: Yale University Press, 1968); and Richard Harris, *A Sacred Trust* (New York: New American Library, 1966).

5. Harris, *supra*, note 4; Theodore Marmor, *The Politics of Medicare*, 2d rev. ed. (Chicago: Aldine, 1973).

6. Oliver Garceau, *The Political Life of the American Medical Association* (Cambridge, MA: Harvard University Press, 1941); *Yale Law Journal*, *supra*, note 1; Rosemary Stevens, *American Medicine and the Public Interest* (New Haven: Yale University Press, 1972); Rayack, *supra*, note 1; and Stanley Kelley, *Professional Public Relations and Political Power* (Baltimore: Johns Hopkins University Press, 1956).

7. Jeanne Brand, *Doctors and the State* (Baltimore: Johns Hopkins University Press, 1965); and Harry Eckstein, *Pressure Group Politics: The Case of the British Medical Association* (Stanford: Stanford University Press, 1960).

8. William Safran, *Veto-Group Politics: The Case of Health Insurance Reform in West Germany* (San Francisco: Chandler, 1967); and Frieder Naschold, *Kassenärzte und Krankenversicherungsreform: Zu einer Theorie der Statuspolitik* (Freiberg im Breisgau: Rombach, 1967).

9. Robin F. Badgley and Samuel Wolfe, *Doctors on Strike* (New York: Atherton, 1967).

10. Theodore Marmor and David Thomas, "The Politics of Paying Physicians: The Determinants of Government Payment Methods in England, Sweden and the United States," *International Journal of Health Services* 1 (January 1971): 71–78; and Theodore Marmor and David Thomas, "Doctors, Politics and Pay Disputes: 'Pressure Group Politics' Revisited," *British Journal of Political Science* 2 (October 1972): 412–42.

11. For an expansion of this argument, see Rayack, *supra*, note 1, chaps. 3–4; Milton Friedman, *Capitalism and Freedom* (Chicago: University of Chicago Press, 1962), pp. 149–60; Reuben Kessel, "The A.M.A. and the Supply of Physicians," *Law and Contemporary Problems* 35 (Spring 1970): 267–83; and Stevens, *supra*, note 6, pp. 55–74 and 348–57.

12. See Rayack, *supra*, note 1, pp. 5–6; and *Yale Law Journal*, *supra*, note 1, pp. 977–80.

13. Rayack, *supra*, note 1, pp. 5–6 and *Yale Law Journal*, *supra*, note 1, pp. 988–97.

14. Kenneth Arrow, "Uncertainty and the Welfare Economics of Medical Care," *American Economic Review* 53 (December 1963): 949–52; Herbert Klarman, *The Economics of Health* (New York: Columbia University Press, 1965), pp. 14–15; and Victor Fuchs, *Who Shall Live?* (New York: Basic Books, 1974), p. 57.

15. For more detailed analyses of the effect of physicians' prices on health service expenditures, see Martin Feldstein, "The Rising Price of Physicians' Services," *Review of Economics and Statistics* 52 (May 1970):

121–33; and Victor Fuchs, "The Basic Forces Influencing the Costs of Medical Care," in Victor Fuchs, ed., *Essays in the Economics of Health and Medical Care* (New York: National Bureau of Economic Research, 1972), pp. 39–50.

16. Talcott Parsons, *The Social System* (New York: Free Press, 1951), pp. 456–57.

17. Mark Field, *Doctor and Patient in Soviet Russia*, Russian Research Center Studies No. 29 (Cambridge, MA: Harvard University Press, 1957), chap. 9, pp. 146–80.

18. Eckstein, *supra*, note 7.

19. Marmor and Thomas, "The Politics of Paying Physicians," *supra*, note 10; and Marmor and Thomas, "Doctors, Politics and Pay Disputes," *supra*, note 10.

20. Marmor and Thomas, "The Politics of Paying Physicians," *supra*, note 10, pp. 72–73.

21. Marmor and Thomas, "Doctors, Politics and Pay Disputes," *supra*, note 10, p. 432.

22. See, for example, Freidson (*supra*, note 2, pp. 12–22) for the argument that the development of a practical, demonstrably effective technology was crucial to the attainment of a professional autonomy. Freidson would in no way argue that technical expertise is a sufficient condition for professional status, but he does emphasize the "monopoly on technique" more than many scholars. Dietrich Ruschmeyer ("Doctors and Lawyers: A Comment on the Theory of Professions," *Canadian Review of Sociology and Anthropology* 1 [1964]: 17–30) explores different aspects of "technical competence" in the medical and legal professions, but also insists that a profession is characterized by the relevance of its technical work to the central values of society. In general, economists tend to emphasize the importance of physicians' technical expertise as an explanation of professional power. They contrast the market position of consumers of medical care with that of consumers of material goods and note that the relatively greater "consumer ignorance" in the medical care market renders physicians particularly powerful. See, for example, Rayack, *supra*, note 1, pp. 4–5; Klarman, *supra*, note 14, pp. 14–15.

23. Most versions of this argument are based on the pioneering work of Talcott Parsons, *supra*, note 16, pp. 428–79.

24. For a fascinating discussion of the development and consequences of this paradigm, see René Dubos, *Mirage of Health* (New York: Harper & Row, 1959), especially chaps. 4 and 5.

25. See, for example, Parsons, *supra*, note 16, p. 450, for a description of the cultural expectation that physicians should "do everything possible" for the patient. In a more recent essay, "Definitions of Health and Illness in the Light of American Values and Social Structure" (E. Gartly Jaco, ed., *Patients, Physicians and Illness*, 2d ed. [New York: Free Press, 1972], pp. 97–117) Parsons relates the interventionist bias of medicine to the general value placed on activism and mastery over the environment in American culture. Freidson (*supra*, note 2, pp. 255–59) reviews several studies that purport to demonstrate physicians' propensity to err on the side of active intervention. Thomas Scheff has analyzed physician behavior from a decision-analytic perspective and suggests that under conditions of uncertainty, "physicians and the public typically overvalue

medical treatment relative to nontreatment as a course of action" ("Decision Rules and Types of Error, and Their Consequences in Medical Diagnosis," *Behavioral Science* 8 [July 1963]: 103). Finally, Ivan Illich has explored the social, political, psychological, and clinical consequences of medical interventionist thinking in *Medical Nemesis: The Expropriation of Health* (London: Calder and Boyers, 1975).

26. Parsons, "Definitions," *supra*, note 25, p. 110.

27. See, for example, Earl Koos, *The Health of Regionville* (New York: Columbia University Press, 1954), pp. 30–38; and David Mechanic, "Response Factors in Illness: The Study of Illness Behavior," *Social Pyschiatry* 1 (1966): 11–20.

28. See Victor Fuchs, *Who Shall Live? supra*, note 14, chap. 2; Katherine Bauer, "Averting the Self-Inflicted Nemeses (Sins) from Dangerous Driving, Smoking, and Drinking," in Selma J. Mushkin, ed., *Consumer Incentives for Health Care* (New York: Prodist, 1974), pp. 3–33; and James W. Vaupel, "Early Death: An American Tragedy," *Law and Contemporary Problems* 40 (1976): 73–121.

29. Harris, *supra*, note 4.

30. For a comprehensive discussion of this point, see Freidson, *supra*, note 2, chaps. 10 and 12.

31. Thomas Szasz, "Malingering: 'Diagnosis' or Social Condemnation?" *AMA Archives of Neurology and Psychiatry* 76 (1956): 432–43.

32. See Robert Martinson, "What Works?—Questions and Answers about Prison Reform," *The Public Interest*, no. 35 (Spring 1974), pp. 22–54.

33. Illich, *supra*, note 25.

34. For an interesting example of selection of paramedical personnel by the communities they serve, see Victor W. Sidel, "The Barefoot Doctors of the People's Republic of China," *New England Journal of Medicine* 286 (June 15, 1972): 1292–1300.

35. The classic exposition of this theory is by David B. Truman, *The Governmental Process* (New York: Knopf, 1959).

36. For some views on the medical profession as a dominant monopoly, see Robert Alford, *Health Care Politics: Ideological and Interest Group Barriers to Reform* (Chicago: University of Chicago Press, 1975); Jeffrey Berlant, *Profession and Monopoly* (Berkeley: University of California Press, 1975); Mark J. Green with Beverly C. Moore, Jr., and Bruce Wasserstein, *The Closed Enterprise System* (New York: Grossman, 1972), pp. 266–69; and Clark C. Havighurst, testimony and materials relating to testimony, in U.S. Senate, *Competition and the Health Services*, Hearings Before the Subcommittee on Antitrust and Monopoly of the Committee on the Judiciary, 93d Cong., 2d sess., May 17, 1972, pt. 2, pp. 1036–89.

37. See, for example, Mancur Olson, *The Logic of Collective Action* (Cambridge, MA: Harvard University Press, 1965); and Albert O. Hirschman, *Exit, Voice and Loyalty* (Cambridge, MA: Harvard University Press, 1970).

38. A very clear exposition of the arguments for and against market controls in health care by an advocate of market control is presented in Havighurst, *supra*, note 36, pp. 1072–76.

39. This problem is discussed very thoroughly and intelligently by Freidson, *supra*, note 2, chaps. 15 and 16.

40. This discussion will exclude care provided under the Medicare and Medicaid programs, the Veterans Administration, the Indian Health Service, military hospitals, and other government programs. The aim here is to provide a description of "mainstream" American medicine, the pattern from which all other patterns of practice have emerged.

41. Freidson, *supra*, note 2, chap. 7, pp. 137–57; Eliot Freidson, *Doctoring Together* (New York: Elsevier, 1975); and Marcia Millman, *The Unkindest Cut* (New York: Morrow, 1977).

42. Freidson, *supra*, note 2, pp. 145–47.

43. Ibid., pp. 149–51.

44. Ibid., pp. 191–200; and Eliot Freidson, *Professional Dominance* (New York: Atherton, 1970), pp. 99–102.

45. Robert Derbyshire, "What Should the Profession Do about the Incompetent Physician?" *Journal of the American Medical Association* 194 (1965); 1288.

46. Robert Derbyshire, *Medical Licensure and Discipline in the United States* (Baltimore: Johns Hopkins University Press, 1969), p. 33.

47. Sometimes licensing boards actually delegate their disciplinary functions to the professional associations. In some cases, the boards rely on the grievance procedures of the associations to initiate disciplinary procedures, and the state may even subsidize the associations. In other cases, the associations actually subsidize the boards. U.S. Department of Health, Education, and Welfare, Office of Assistant Secretary for Health and Scientific Affairs, *Report on Licensure and Related Health Personnel Credentialing*, DHEW Publication No. (HSM)72–11, June 1971, pp. 31–32.

48. For a useful description of this and other obstacles to more effective self-discipline, see Robert C. Derbyshire, "Medical Ethics and Discipline," *Journal of the American Medical Association* 288 (April 1974): 59–62.

49. American Medical Association, Law Division, *Disciplinary Digest: Court Decisions in Regard to Disciplinary Actions by State Boards of Medical Examiners* (1967), p. 16.

50. Ibid., pp. 7–8; and see also State Board of Medical Examiners v. Weiler, 402 p.2d 606 (Colo. 1965), cited therein.

51. Robert C. Derbyshire, interview in *American Medical News* 18 (October 6, 1975): 11, col. 1.

52. See David W. Louisell and Harold Williams, *Medical Malpractice*, 2 vols. with annual supplements (Albany: Bender, 1973), vol. 1, paragraph 8.04; and Allen H. McCoid, "The Care Required of Medical Practitioners," *Vanderbilt Law Journal* 12 (June 1959): 549–632, esp. 558–60.

53. Comment, "Standard of Care for Medical Practitioners— Abandonment of the Locality Rule," *Kentucky Law Journal* 60 (Fall 1971): 209–16.

54. U.S. Department of Health, Education, and Welfare, *Medical Malpractice: Report of the Secretary's Commission on Medical Malpractice*, DHEW Publication No. (OS)73–88, January 16, 1973, pp. 42–43.

55. One study of physicians' attitude toward the malpractice situation found, in fact, that physicians who had been "touched by malpractice" (i.e., sued or threatened) were more likely than a control group to blame the malpractice situation on causes outside the profession, such as "aggressive lawyers," "declining public regard for physicians," or "increasing public education," than on causes within the profession, such as

"poor communication between physician and patient," "increasing complexity of medical practice," "bad medicine," or "poorly trained physicians." See William Pabst, "A Medical Opinion Survey of Physicians' Attitudes on Medical Malpractice," in ibid., appendix, pp. 83–86.

56. See Eli P. Bernzweig, "Defensive Medicine," in U.S. Department of HEW, *supra*, note 55, appendix, pp. 38–40.

57. A very useful compilation of data on the malpractice crisis is American Medical Association, "Malpractice in Focus," Source Document prepared by the editors of *Prism*, August 1975.

Chapter Two

1. See Theodore S. Hamerow, *The Social Foundations of German Unification 1858–1871: Ideas and Institutions* (Princeton, NJ: Princeton University Press, paperback ed., 1969), pp. 181–221; and Gaston V. Rimlinger, *Welfare Policy and Industrialization in Europe, America, and Russia* (New York: Wiley, 1971), pp. 89–98. Rimlinger provides an excellent history of the development of German social insurance in chap. 4.

2. Alexander Gerschenkron, *Bread and Democracy in Germany*, 2d ed. (New York: Fertig, 1966; 1st ed., Berkeley: University of California Press, 1943).

3. Ralf Dahrendorf, *Society and Democracy in Germany* (Garden City: Doubleday, Anchor Books, 1969), p. 37.

4. Ibid., pp. 36–37.

5. Guido Goldman, "The German Political System," in S. B. Beer and A. Ulam, eds., *Patterns of Government* (New York: Random House, 1973), p. 478.

6. Harry Pross, *Die Zerstörung der Deutschen Politik* (Frankfurt, 1959), p. 360, cited in Dahrendorf, *supra*, note 3, p. 59.

7. For an analysis of the political motivations of Disraeli's programs, see Samuel H. Beer, *British Politics in the Collectivist Age* (New York: Random House, Vintage Books, 1969), pp. 245–76.

8. The description of accident insurance legislation is based on Rimlinger, *supra*, note 1, pp. 112–20.

9. Otto Quandt, *Die Anfänge der Bismarckschen Sozialgesetzgebung* (Berlin: Ebering, 1938), p. 25, cited in Rimlinger, *supra*, note 1, p. 118.

10. Hamerow, *supra*, note 1, pp. 211–13.

11. Rimlinger, *supra*, note 1, pp. 126–27.

12. Heinz Ströer, *Die Soziale Krankenversicherung* (Munich: C. H. Beck, 1971), pp. 74–75.

13. For a more detailed explication of membership and eligibility requirements, see *ibid.*, pp. 74–89; and Bundesminister für Arbeit und Sozialordnung (BMA), *Übersicht über die Soziale Sicherung 1977* (Bonn, 1977), pp. 184–90.

14. BMA, *supra*, note 13, p. 184.

15. BMA, "Statistische Daten zur konzertierte Aktion im Gesundheitswesen," Bonn, 28 February 1978, table 7a. Figures are for 1976.

16. See especially Andrew Schonfeld, *Modern Capitalism* (London: Oxford University Press, 1965), chap. 11.

17. Goldman, *supra*, note 5, pp. 574–75.

18. Lewis J. Edinger, *Politics in Germany: Attitudes and Processes* (Boston: Little, Brown, 1968), p. 302.

19. Renate Mayntz and Fritz Scharpf, *Policymaking in the German Federal Bureaucracy* (Amsterdam: Elsevier, 1975), pp. 135–36 and 156–57; and Safran, *supra*, chap. 1, note 8, pp. 34–35.

20. Mayntz and Scharpf, *supra*, note 19, p. 136. The rules governing the conduct of ministries are the *Gemeinsame Geschäftsordnungen der Bundesministerium*.

21. Ibid., pp. 136 and 157–63.

22. Safran, *supra*, chap. 1, note 8, p. 212.

23. Dahrendorf (*supra*, note 3) argues: "It is the rationale of all state-inaugurated social policy of the European type to immobilize people by providing for them at the place at which they happen to be, until their dying day and thus make it unnecessary for them to act rationally, that is, to explore the market of life chances themselves" (p. 47). But while it is true that German social insurance did have as a goal the binding of workers to their employers, this need not be true of all social insurance programs. So long as benefits are made portable, and so long as *all* employers are required to provide the same social benefits, a state social insurance program does not weaken the incentive to search out the best employment possibilities.

The reason the original health insurance program did restrict labor mobility is precisely that it was not universal—it did not apply to all employers, nor did it apply to all types of jobs. Under the current system, which is nearly universal, national health insurance cannot be said to be a market restricting force.

Chapter Three

1. Freidson, *supra*, chap. 1, note 2, pp. 72–73.

2. See, for example, William J. Goode, "Encroachment, Charlatanism and the Emerging Profession: Psychology, Sociology and Medicine," *American Sociological Review* 25 (December 1960): 902–14; William J. Goode, "The Librarian: From Occupation to Profession?" *Library Quarterly* 31 (October 1961): 306–18; Ernest Greenwood, "Attributes of a Profession," *Social Work* 2 (July 1957): 44–55; and Theodore Caplow, *The Sociology of Work* (Minneapolis: University of Minnesota Press, 1954), pp. 139–40.

3. See Everett C. Hughes, "The Professions in Society," *Canadian Journal of Economics and Political Science* 26 (February 1960): 54–60; T. H. Marshall, "The Recent History of Professionalism in Relation to Social Structure and Social Policy," *Canadian Journal of Economics and Political Science* 5 (August 1939): 325–40.

4. Magali Sarfatti Larson, *The Rise of Professionalism: A Sociological Analysis* (Berkeley: University of California Press, 1977).

5. This is the central thesis of Dahrendorf, *supra*, chap. 2, note 3.

6. Paul Lüth, *Niederlassung und Praxis: Eine kritische Einführung* (Stuttgart: Georg Thieme, 1969), p. 57; and Theodor Plaut, *Der Gewerkschaftskampf der Deutschen Ärzte*, Volkswirtschaftliche Abhandlungen der badischen Hochschulen, Heft 14 (Karlsrühe: G. Braunsche, 1913), p. 25, note 2.

7. Christa Rauskolb, *Lobby in Weiss* (Frankfurt: Europaische Verlags-

anstalt, 1976), pp. 162–63; William Safran, *supra*, chap. 1, note 8, p. 107; and Plaut, *supra*, note 6, pp. 32–35.

8. L. Ebermayer, *Arzt und Patient in der Rechtsprechung*, 3d and 4th eds., 1925, cited by Lüth, *supra*, note 6, p. 66.

9. Lüth, *supra*, note 6, p. 66.

10. Heinz Schmitt, *Entstehung und Wandlungen der Zielsetzungen, der Struktur und der Wirkungen der Berufsverbände* (Berlin: Duncker und Humblot, 1966), pp. 27–29; and Plaut, *supra*, note 6, pp. 19–21.

11. Plaut, *supra*, note 6, p. 20.

12. Schmitt, *supra*, note 10, p. 28.

13. Ibid., pp. 30–31.

14. Ibid., p. 32.

15. Ibid., p. 36; and Plaut, *supra*, note 6, pp. 24–26.

16. Schmitt, *supra*, note 10, pp. 37–38; Plaut's membership figures for 1894 are slightly, but not significantly, different—245 associations representing 64 percent of all physicians. Plaut, *supra*, note 6, p. 28.

17. Schmitt, *supra*, note 10, p. 44.

18. See Bundesärzteordnung, 1970, in *Bundesgesetzblatt 1*: 237.

19. Schmitt, *supra*, note 10, p. 43.

20. Plaut, *supra*, note 6, p. 67.

21. Ibid., pp. 61–62.

22. Ibid., p. 61.

23. The following information on contract commissions is from Plaut, *supra*, note 6, pp. 36–43.

24. Schmitt, *supra*, note 10, pp. 46–47.

25. Plaut, *supra*, note 6, p. 31.

26. Schmitt, *supra*, note 10, p. 48.

27. The following description of the "Landmann system" is taken from his own work, F. Landmann, *Die Lösung der Kassenarztfrage* (Elberfeld: Grimpe, 1898), and especially his model contract for physicians attached to a polyclinic, pp. 53–56.

28. Plaut, *supra*, note 6, pp. 87–88.

29. The full text of Dr. Hartmann's letter can be found in Plaut, *supra*, note 6, pp. 90–94.

30. Schmitt, *supra*, note 10, pp. 38 and 58.

31. Ibid., pp. 59–62.

32. Ibid., pp. 56, 63–64.

33. Plaut, *supra*, note 6, p. 129.

34. Ibid., pp. 138 and 144.

35. Ibid., p. 143.

36. Schmitt, *supra*, note 10, p. 73.

37. Calculated from data in ibid., p. 77.

38. Deutsche Ärztevereinsbund, *Ärztliches Vereinsblatt für Deutschland*, 1879, p. 98, cited in Naschold, *supra*, chap. 1, note 8, p. 47.

39. Naschold, *supra*, chap. 1, note 8, pp. 46–47.

40. Plaut, *supra*, note 6, p. 68.

41. Schmitt, *supra*, note 10, p. 78.

42. Felix Meyer, *Zur Frage der freie Arztwahl* (Hamburg: 1904), cited in Plaut, *supra*, note 6, p. 161.

43. Rauskolb, *supra*, note 7, pp. 121–22.

44. H. D. Goldammer, "Die Beziehungen zwischen Kassenärztlichen Vereinigungen und Krankenkassen," Dissertation, Cologne; 1964, p. 19, cited in Rauskolb, *supra*, note 7, p. 123.

45. Ibid., p. 123; and Naschold, *supra*, chap. 1, note 8, pp. 57–59.

46. Following the centralizing trend of the National Socialist government, the authority to conclude contracts with sickness funds was transferred to the National Association of Insurance Doctors in 1933; after the end of World War II, the power was transferred back to the regional associations.

47. Actually, when the concept of a fixed ratio was first introduced in the Berlin Treaty, the ratio was treated as a minimum criterion. The emergency order of 1923 raised the ratio to 1:1,000, but treated the ratio as a maximum criterion. The order of 1931 raised the ratio once again, to 1:600, but treated it as a "guideline". Naschold, *supra*, chap. 1, note 8, pp. 59–60. Since the ratio was between doctors and fund members, not including dependents, the actual ratio of doctors to insured persons was much lower, probably 1:2,000.

48. Naschold, *supra*, chap. 1, note 8, p. 60; and L. Richter, *Das Kassenarztrecht von 1931/32* (Leipzig, 1932), pp. 63 ff, cited in Rauskolb, *supra*, note 7, p. 126.

Chapter Four

1. Statistisches Bundesamt, *Statistisches Jahrbuch für die Bundesrepublik Deutschland, 1978* (Stuttgart: Kohlhammer, 1978), table 17.10.

2. Wissenschaftliches Institut der Ortskrankenkassen, Seminar zur kassenärztlichen Bedarfsplanung, *Die Verteilung der niedergelassenen Ärzte und Zahnärzte in der Bundesrepublik Deutschland und die Entwicklungstrends* (Bad Godesberg: Bundesverband der Ortskrankenkassen, n.d.). Figures are for 1974.

3. Romuald Schicke, *Arzt und Gesundheitsversorgung im gesellschaftlichen Sicherungssystem* (Freiburg: Rombach, 1971).

4. J. Cremer, *Grundlagen der ärztlichen Rechts- und Berufskunde* (Stuttgart, 1962), p. 44; cited in Schicke, *supra*, note 3, p. 84.

5. American Medical Association, *Profile of Medical Practice 1978* (Chicago, 1978), p. 144.

6. Safran, *supra*, chap. 1, note 8, pp. 115–16.

7. Schicke, *supra*, note 3, p. 90.

8. Wolfgang Wekel, "Änderungen des Kassenarztrechts," *Die Ortskrankenkasse* 59 (February 15, 1977): 117; and RVO 368c, paragraph 3, as amended by the Gesetz zur Weiterentwicklung des Kassenarztrechts, December 28, 1976 (*Bundesgesetzblatt* 2: 3,871).

9. Gesellschaft für Sozialen Fortschritt e. V., (GSF), *Der Wandel der Stellung des Arztes im Einkommensgefüge* (Bonn, 1974), p. 19.

10. Ibid., table 14, p. 45.

11. Naschold, *supra*, chap. 1, note 8, p. 139.

12. *Die Ortskrankenkasse* 58 (1976): 500–501.

13. Schicke, *supra*, note 3, p. 86.

14. Berufs- und Facharztordnung 32 Abs. 2 u.3, cited in Josef Daniels and Manfred Bulling, *Bundesärzteordnung; Kommentar* (Berlin, 1963), p. 400, in Schicke, *supra*, note 3, p. 86.

15. Schicke, *supra*, note 3, pp. 143–44.

16. GSF, *supra*, note 9, p. 75. Most of the 2,238 group practices in

1978 were composed of two doctors in the same family, and about 780 were simply arrangements for sharing laboratory services only. Ulrich Geissler, personal communication.

17. Schicke, *supra*, note 3, p. 143.

18. These figures count the physician as part of "personnel." GSF, *supra*, note 9, p. 74; and Uwe Reinhardt, "Health Costs and Expenditures in the Federal Republic of Germany and the United States," in Teh-wei Hu, ed., *International Health Costs and Expenditures*, DHEW Publication No. (NIH)76–1067 (1976), p. 254.

19. GSF, *supra*, note 9, p. 74.

20. Schicke, *supra*, note 3, p. 143.

21. GSF, *supra*, note 9, p. 77.

22. Ibid., pp. 74–76.

23. See especially Victor Fuchs and Marcia J. Kramer, *Determinants of Expenditures for Physicians' Services in the United States 1948–1968*, National Center for Health Services Research and Development, Department of Health Education and Welfare, DHEW Publication No. (HSM)73–3013 (December 1972); and A. C. Higgins, "Two-Thirds of a Medical Equation: Pathology and Patients," in Irwin Deutscher and Elizabeth Thompson, eds., *Among the People* (New York: Basic Books, 1968), pp. 279–93.

24. Milton Roemer and M. Shain, *Hospital Utilization under Insurance* (Chicago: American Hospital Association, 1959); Martin Feldstein, "Hospital Cost Inflation: A Study of Non-Profit Price Dynamics," *American Economic Review* 61 (1971): 853–72.

25. Theo Siebeck, "Das Vergütungssystem im Kassenarztrecht," *Die Ortskrankenkasse* 45 (1963): 512.

26. Fritz Kastner, "Kassenärztliche Vergütungssysteme—Pauschal- oder Einzelleistungsvergütung?" *Die Ortskrankenkasse* 47 (1965): 57.

27. "Physician's assistant" is used here not in the American sense of licensed paramedical personnel, but rather simply as a designation for any office help used by a physician. Nonphysician health professionals (e.g., laboratory technicians, physical therapists) may be reimbursed under social insurance only when their services are ordered by a physician or when they work under supervision of a physician. See BMA, *Übersicht über die Soziale Sicherung 1974* (Bonn, 1974), p. 165.

28. See Judith Lorber, "Deviance as Performance: The Case of Illness," in Eliot Freidson and Judith Lorber, eds., *Medical Men and Their Work* (Chicago: Aldine, 1972), pp. 414–22; Deborah Stone, "Physicians as Gatekeepers: Illness Certification as a Rationing Device," *Public Policy* 27 (Spring 1979): 227–54.

29. Reichsversicherungsordnung, section 181.

30. Deutscher Bundestag, 7. Wahlperiode, *Bericht der Bundesregierung über die Erfahrung mit der Einführung von Maßnahmen zur Früherkennung von Krankheiten als Pflichtleistungen der Krankenkassen sowie den zusätzlich von den Krankenkassen gewährten Maßnahmen der Vorsorgenhilfe*, Drucksache 7/454, April 5, 1973, pp. 28–30.

31. Ibid. table 9, p. 34.

32. Personal interview, August 21, 1973.

Chapter Five

1. John Kenneth Galbraith, *American Capitalism: The Concept of Coun-*

tervailing Power (Boston: Houghton Mifflin, 1952), especially pp. 108–34.

2. See Charles H. Hesson, *John Kenneth Galbraith and His Critics* (New York: New American Library, 1972), pp. 41–63, for a review of the critiques.

3. Philipp Herder-Dorneich, *Analyse der Gesetzlichen Krankenversicherung* (Berlin: Erich Schmidt, 1965), pp. 109–26.

4. See Michael Polanyi, *The Great Transformation* (New York: Rinehart, 1944; repr. ed., Boston: Beacon, 1957); and Charles E. Lindblom, *Politics and Markets* (New York: Basic Books, 1977).

5. Bundesministerium für Jugend, Familie und Gesundheit, *Gesundheitsbericht (Bonn, 1971), p. 158.* Even more significant than private expenditures are those by public health agencies, pension authorities, and accident insurance authorities for health services, as well as public subsidies to hospitals.

6. George von Haunalter and Virginia V. Chandler, "Health Care Expenditures in Four Western European Countries," SRI Business Intelligence Program, Research Report No. 606 (Menlo Park, CA: Stanford Research Institute, 1978), p. 5.

7. BMA, *supra*, chap. 2, note 13, p. 196.

8. See Horst Ruegenberg, "Perspektiven einer Weiterentwicklung der Gesetzlichen Krankenversicherung," *Die Ortskrankenkasse* 58 (January 1976): 12–24; and GSF, *supra*, chap. 4, note 9, pp. 43–44.

9. *Die Ortskrankenkasse* 58 (April 1, 1976): 259.

10. Ruegenberg, *supra*, note 8, pp. 23–24.

11. *Die Ortskrankenkasse* 58 (March 15, 1976): 211.

12. Ströer, *supra*, chap. 2, note 12, p. 109.

13. Bundesverband der Ortskrankenkassen, "Statistischer Vierteljahresbericht: Die Ortskrankenkassen im Jahre 1977" (Bonn-Bad Godesberg, 1978), table 3. Whether the relative advantages of substitute funds are due to deliberate selection of members or to historical circumstances is a matter of debate among West German analysts.

14. This description of sickness fund self-government is based on BMA, *supra*, chap. 4, note 27, pp. 325–28.

15. Franz-Xaver Kaufmann, Friedhart Hegner, Lutz Hoffmann, and Jürgen Krüger, "Zum Verhältnis zwischen Sozialversicherungsträgern und Versicherten," Forschungsvorhaben im Auftrage des Bundesministeriums für Arbeit und Sozialordnung (Bielefeld, December 1971), pp. 175–76.

16. Instutut für angewandte Sozialforschung (INFAS), "Selbstverwaltung in der Sozialversicherung" (Bonn-Bad Godesberg, July 1975), tables 14, 16, 17, 21, and 22.

17. Berufsbildungsgesetz, August 14, 1969, (*Bundesgesetzblatt* 1:1,112; amended March 12, 1971, *Bundesgesetzblatt* 1:185.

18. The essence of the new law is described in Bundesverband der Ortskrankenkassen, *Geschäftsbericht 1971* (Bonn-Bad Godesberg, 1971), pp. 107–9. A detailed description of the educational curriculum and examinations for social insurance administrative specialists can be found in Bundesverband der Ortskrankenkassen, *Geschäftsbericht 1972* (Bonn-Bad Godesberg, 1972), pp. 109–15.

19. Philipp Herder-Dorneich, *Sozialökonomischer Grundriss der Gesetzlichen Krankenversicherung* (Stuttgart: Kohlhammer, 1966), p. 231.

20. BMA, *supra*, chap. 4, note 27, p. 326.

21. Ralf Dahrendorf, *supra*, chap. 2, note 3, p. 316, for pre-1949 data; Statistisches Bundesamt, *Statistiches Jahrbuch für die Bundesrepublik Deutschland 1974*, p. 127, for post-1949 data.

22. Edinger, *supra*, chap. 2, note 18, p. 211.

23. Kaufmann, et al., *supra*, note 15, p. 160.

24. Institut für angewandte Sozialforschung, *supra*, note 16, p.2.

25. Kaufmann, et al., *supra*, note 15, pp. 119–51; and Herder-Dorneich, *supra*, note 19, pp. 218–22.

26. See *Soziale Sicherung in der Bundesrepublik Deutschland: Bericht der Sozialenquête-Kommission* (Stuttgart: Kohlhammer, 1966), p. 105; Herder-Dorneich, *supra*, note 19, pp. 230–31; and Safran, *supra*, chap. 1, note 8, p. 129.

27. Herder-Dorneich, *supra*, note 19, pp. 233–34.

28. These exceptions are described more fully in BMA, *supra*, chap. 2, note 13, pp. 204–6.

29. BMA, *Arbeits- und Sozialstatistik*, no. 5/6, (1978), p. 185.

30. See Peter Rosenberg, "Die Finanzen der Gesetzlichen Krankenversicherung," *Vierteljahreshefte zur Wirtschaftsforschung* no. 3 (1973), pp. 198–201.

31. BMA, *supra*, chap. 2, note 13, p. 205.

32. GSF, *supra*, chap. 4, note 9, p. 40.

33. *Soziale Sicherung in der Bundesrepublik Deutschland*, *supra*, note 26, p. 204.

34. Ibid., p. 228.

35. GSF, *supra*, note 8, p. 43.

36. "Spiegel-Umfrage: Die Ärzte verlangen zuviel," *Der Spiegel* 31, no. 12 (1977), p. 65.

37. See Dr. Walter Auerbach, "Doppelstandard in der medizinischen Versorgung?" *Sozialer Fortschritt*, no. 2 (1972), pp. 36–38; and Alfred Schmitt, "Medizinische Versorgung muss klassenlos sein!" *Sozialer Fortschritt*, no. 9 (1972), pp. 201–4.

Chapter Six

1. Further detail on both historical and current methods of determining the pool is available in the following: Siebeck, *supra*, chap. 4, note 25, pp. 501–16; Theo Siebeck, "Die Kassenärztliche Gesamtvergütung," *Die Ortskrankenkasse* 47 (1965), 3 pts.: 169–74, 204–11, and 234–41; and Karl Dieter Kortmann, "Der Übergang von der Pauschal- zur Einzelleistungsvergütung bei der Honorierung von kassenärztlichen Leistungen," Doctoral dissertation, Wirtschafts- und Sozialwissenschaftlichen Fakultät, Universität Köln, 1968.

2. Siebeck, *supra*, chap. 4, note 25, pp. 503–4.

3. Theo Siebeck, "Wandlungen und Tendenzen im Kassenarztrecht," *Die Ortskrankenkasse* 53 (1972): 806.

4. Kortmann, *supra*, note 1, pp. 42–43.

5. Siebeck, *supra*, note 1, pp. 205–6; and GSF, *supra*, chap. 4, note 9, pp. 92–93.

6. The various arguments are well summarized in Kastner, *supra*, chap. 4, note 26, 3 pts., pp. 11–16, 57–60, and 89–93.

7. Theo Siebeck, "Vertrags- und Vergütungssystem im Kas-

senarztrecht," cited in Kastner, *supra*, note 6, p. 58.

8. Kastner, *supra*, chap. 4, note 26, p. 12.

9. Ibid., p. 14.

10. See Kortmann, *supra*, note 1, pp. 78–92. Even Siebeck, who years earlier foresaw the difficulties that a fee-for-service payment method would create for cost control, made this same argument in his essays on the cost-control problem in 1976 (*Zur Kostenentwicklung in der Krankenversicherung* [Bonn: Verlag der Ortskrankenkassen, 1976], p. 63).

11. Kastner, *supra*, chap. 4, note 26, p. 15.

12. Ibid., p. 91.

13. Herder-Dorneich, *supra*, chap. 5, note 19, p. 289.

14. See Siebeck, *supra*, note 1, p. 169; and GSF, *supra*, chap. 4, note 9, pp. 89–90.

15. GSF, *supra*, chap. 4, note 9, p. 65.

16. Gustav W. Heinemann, Rolf Leibold, and Peter J. Heinemann, *Kassenarztrecht auf Grund der gesetzlichen Bestimmungen und der Rechtsprechung*, vol. 1, 4th rev. ed., (Berlin and Wiesbaden: Engel-Verlag, 1973), p. I–29i, sec. 18.

17. Lüth, *supra*, chap. 3, note 6, p. 109, and personal interviews.

18. *Bewertungsmaßstab-Ärzte*, Gebührenordnung für die Abrechnung Kassenärztliche Leistungen als Anlage zum Bundesmantelvertrag-Ärzte, July 1, 1973.

19. For a discussion of this problem from the point of view of the sickness funds, see Siebeck, *supra*, note 1, pp. 234 ff.

20. *Der Spiegel* 31, no. 28 (1977), p. 138.

21. Ulrich Geissler, "Ergebnisse der 'Kostenstrukturerhebung für ärztliche und zahnärztliche Praxen 1975' des Statistischen Bundesamtes," Beratungsunterlage Nr. 1066 zum Tagesordnungspunkt II/7 der Vorstandssitzung am 14. September, 1977, Bundesverband der Ortskrankenkassen, Bad Godesberg, mimeo, p. 7.

22. *Der Spiegel*, *supra*, note 20, p. 141. Recently there has been even more concern about overinvestment in and excess use of laboratory equipment.

23. GSF, *supra*, chap. 4, note 9, p. 51; and Thomas Sörenson, "Automatisierte Laborleistungen neu bewertet," *Die Ersatzkasse* 7–8 (1973): 308–12.

Chapter Seven

1. Erwin Liek, cited in Kastner, *supra*, chap. 4, note 26, p. 58.

2. Siebeck, *supra*, chap. 4, note 25, pp. 502–3.

3. Ibid., p. 510.

4. Heinemann, et al., *supra*, chap. 6, note 16, sec. I–29–i, pt. 18.

5. Ibid., sec. I–27–o.

6. Siebeck, *supra*, chap. 4, note 25, p. 510.

7. Heinemann, et al., *supra*, chap. 6, note 16, sec. I–27–o to I–28–b.

8. Siebeck, *supra*, chap. 6, note 3, p. 808.

9. Ibid.

10. Bundessozialgericht, Urteil 6 RKa 15/64, 17. January 1965, cited in E. Üblich, "Zur Prüfung der Wirtschaftlichkeit der kassenärztlichen Leistungen," *Der Niedergelassene Arzt*, no. 2, (1974), p. 11.

11. The following description of economic monitoring comes from two published sources as well as a number of interviews with persons in various AIDs and sickness funds. The published sources are Üblich, *supra*, note 10, two parts, no. 2, pp. 11–22 and no. 3, pp. 75–88 (also published in *Der Kassenarzt*, nos. 5 and 6, 1973); and Bayerischen Landesärztekammer, *Kassenärztliches Praxis–Lexicon*, Anhang 2, "Zur Prüfung der Wirtschaftlichkeit der kassenärztlichen Tätigkeit" (Dachau: Hans Zauner, 1973).

12. Üblich, *supra*, note 10, p. 12.

13. "Case" here means *Behandlungsfall*, which is equivalent to all the services rendered one patient during the accounting quarter. It does not refer to a discrete illness episode, but rather, to one "certificate of insurance" or voucher (*Krankenschein*).

14. Lüth (*supra*, chap. 3, note 6, p. 114) gives a figure of 20–70 percent; Üblich (*supra*, note 11, p. 85) gives a figure of 20–60 percent. One head of a monitoring department said the number of physicians selected for review by the committee in his region was only 5 percent.

15. Üblich (*supra*, note 11, p. 85) estimates 5–10 percent; other estimates are from personal interviews.

16. Üblich (*supra*, note 11, p. 88) gives a figure of 2 to 3.5 percent. GSF, *supra*, chap. 4, note 9, p. 54, gives a figure of 0.5 percent. Other estimates are from personal interviews.

17. Even rarer are cases of revocation of a permit for persistent *under-provision* of care, but they do occasionally happen.

18. Lüth, *supra*, chap. 3, note 6, p. 105.

19. Üblich, *supra*, chap. note 11, p. 75.

20. See Urteil des Landessozialgerichts Rheinland-Pfalz, 13. 11. 72. (L KA 1/72), cited in *Münchner Medizinische Wochenschrift* 116, no. 43 (1974): 34; and Üblich, *supra*, note 11, p. 12.

21. Peter Rosenberg, "Kontrolle der Kostenentwicklung im Gesundheitswesen," *Sozialer Fortschritt* nos. 7/8 (1974): 166; and Rosenberg, *supra*, chap. 5, note 30, p. 204.

22. The American curves are based on 1949 data and the German curves on 1963 data, simply because those years are the only ones for which appropriate data were available. The time difference does not weaken the point, however, since the argument is that economic monitoring alters the income distribution in comparison with what it would be under an unregulated market system. Some factors that should be taken into consideration, however, are the extent of specialization within the profession and the distribution of physicians among various sized communities, because both specialization and practice in a large community are correlated with higher incomes for American physicians. Income inequality among American physicians diminished between 1941 and 1949 at least partly because of increasing urbanization. Since the West German medical profession has always been relatively less specialized than the American, one would guess that the gap between the Lorenz curves would be even greater if controls for degree of specialization were introduced. See George J. Stiegler, *Trends in Employment in the Service Industries*, National Bureau of Economic Research Studies No. 59 (Princeton: Princeton University Press, 1956), pp. 131–32.

23. See Dr. Gerhard Martin, "Warum die Kassenärztliche Versorg-

ung nicht wirtschaftlicher werden kann?" *Medical Tribune* (West German ed.) 12, no. 26 (July 1, 1977), pp. 21—22.

24. See B. Schneider, "Probleme der statistischen Analyse der kassenärztlichen Abrechnungen," Abteilung für Biometrie und Medizinische Informatik der Medizinischen Hochschule Hannover, mimeo, 1977.

25. See Murray Edelman, *The Symbolic Uses of Politics* (Urbana, Ill.: University of Illinois Press, 1964).

26. I am grateful to Manfred Pflanz for pointing out this aspect of the symbolic function of economic monitoring.

Chapter Eight

1. Although a blue-collar worker was nominally entitled to only 65% of net earnings, supplements for dependents could often raise a worker's wage continuation payments to a level *above* his after-tax net earnings.

2. The best English-language description of wage continuation payments as a political issue is Safran, *supra*, chap. 1, note 8.

3. A useful compilation of articles on the Law of Wage Continuation Payments is the special symposium issue of *Die Ortskrankenkasse* 51 (December 1 and 15, 1969).

4. In the American literature, see especially Koos, *supra*, chap. 1, note 27, pp. 30–38. In German, see especially Christian von Ferber, *Sozialpolitik in der Wohlstandsgesellschaft* (Hamburg: Christian Wegner, 1967); and Walter Zimmermann, *Fehlzeiten und industrieller Konflikt* (Stuttgart: Enke, 1970).

5. See Mark V. Pauly, "The Economics of Moral Hazard: Comment," *American Economic Review* 58 (June 1968): 531–36.

6. Deutscher Bundestag, 6. Wahlperiode, *Bericht über die Erfahrung mit der Begutachtung der Arbeitsunfähigkeit durch den Vertrauensärztlichen Dienst (VäD) und über das Zusammenwirken der Kassenärzte (Kassenzahnärzte), der Krankenkassen und das VäD*, Drucksache VI/3200, February 23, 1972, p. 12. (Hereafter cited as *VäD Bericht.*)

7. Verordnung des Reichspräsidenten zur Behebung finanzieller, wirtschaftlicher und sozialer Notstände vom 26. Juli 1930, *Reichsgesetzblatt* 1: 311, 325, cited in ibid., sec. 18.

8. *VäD Bericht, supra*, note 6, sec. 22–35.

9. Reichsversicherungsordnung, sec. 369b.

10. See *VäD Bericht, supra*, note 6, appendix C.

11. Ibid., p. 22, table 3.

12. *Soziale Sicherung in der Bundesrepublik Deutschland: Bericht der Sozialenquête-Kommission, supra*, chap. 5, note 26, p. 215.

13. *VäD Bericht, supra*, note 6, sec. 54.

14. Ibid., appendix C, tables 1–3.

15. Ibid., p. 22.

16. See generally Safran, *supra*, chap. 1, note 8.

17. Herder-Dorneich, *supra*, chap. 5, note 19, pp. 45–48.

18. The estimates are only rough, but do illustrate the dramatic reduction in the proportion of certificates summoned after 1970. Estimates for 1969 are based on data in *VäD Bericht, supra*, note 6, appendix C, tables 3 and 6; and Hans Hartwig, "Aufgaben des Vertrauensärztlichen

Dienstes," *Die Ortskrankenkasse* 52 (September 1, 1970): 570. Estimates for 1971 are based on data in *VäD Bericht*, tables 3, 3a, 8, and 10.

19. Hartwig, *supra*, note 18.

20. This theoretical analysis of the deterrence effect is also supported by the cross-regional data in Sven Günther, "Beeinflussung des Krankenstandes durch den Vertrauensärztlichen Dienst," *Bundesarbeitsblatt* 14 (July 10, 1963): 431–33.

21. See *VäD Bericht*, *supra*, note 6, pp. 20–21.

22. Günther, *supra*, note 20, p. 431.

23. *VäD Bericht*, *supra*, note 6, p. 32.

Chapter Nine

1. BMA, *supra*, chap. 2, note 15, table 10.

2. Haunalter and Chandler, *supra*, chap. 5, note 6.

3. U.S. Department of Health, Education, and Welfare, *Health: United States, 1978*, DHEW Publication No. (PHS) 78–1232, 1978, table 148, p. 382.

4. Haunalter and Chandler, *supra*, chap. 5, note 6, p. 5. (Percentages were calculated by the author from absolute figures.)

5. Calculated from BMA, *supra*, chap. 2, note 15, table 9.

6. Estimate for West German office-based physicians is from Statistisches Bundesamt, Fachserie 2, Unternehmen und Arbeitsstätten, Reihe 1.6.1, "Kostenstruktur bei Ärzten, Zahnärzten, Tierärzten 1975." United States figure is from Zachary Dyckman, *A Study of Physicians' Fees* (Washington, DC: Council on Wage and Price Stability, 1978), p. 75. For the comparison of American and West German doctors' incomes, the conversion from Deutschmarks to dollars was made using an exchange rate of DM 2.3 per dollar, which approximates the prevailing rate in 1975.

The German figure represents a *mean* net income, and the American figure represents the *median* net income, so the difference between the two countries is apt to be slightly overstated.

7. U.S. figures are from Dyckman, *supra*, note 6, p. 75, and are based on the *median* net income of non-salaried, office-based physicians. West German figures are calculated from *mean* net income before taxes for office-based physicians (DM149, 247) given in Statistisches Bundesamt, *supra*, note 6, and an average wage and salary (DM 22, 426) given in BMA *supra*, chap. 2, note 15, table 12. Again, the apparent difference is apt to be slightly overstated.

8. GSF, *supra*, chap. 4, note 9, pp. 21–22.

9. See ibid., pp. 68–71; Rosenberg, *supra*, chap. 7, note 21, p. 168; and Wirtschafts- und Sozialwissenchaftliches Institut des Deutschen Gewerkschaftsbundes GmbH (WSI), *Die Gesundheitssicherung in der Bundesrepublik Deutschland: Analyse und Vorschläge zur Reform,* 2d ed. (Köln: Bund Verlag, 1971), p. 69.

10. GSF, *supra*, chap. 4, note 9, p. 40.

11. Ibid., p. 53; Siebeck, *supra* chap. 6, note 10, pp. 64–66.

12. "Empfehlungsvereinbarung zur Gesamtvergütung," *Die Ortskrankenkasse* 58 (May 1976): 345–46. See also Heinz Bluthmann, "Deckel auf dem Topf," *Die Zeit*, May 14, 1976, p. 16.

13. BMA *supra*, chap. 2, note 15, table 11.

14. The text of the law can be found in the *Bundesgesetzblatt*, June 30, 1977, pp. 1069–85. Sources for the description below are: Deutscher Bundestag, *Sozialbericht 1978 der Bundesregierung*, 8. Wahlperiode, Drucksache 8/1805, May 12, 1978, pp. 26–32; and BMA, *Eine stabile Rentenversicherung und eine gesunde Krankenversicherung* (Bonn, 1977). A more comprehensive review of the Health Care Cost Containment Act of 1977 can be found in Deborah Stone, "Health Care Cost Containment in West Germany," *Journal of Health Politics, Policy and Law* 4 (1979): 176–99.

15. See Arnold J. Heidenheimer and Donald P. Kommers, *The Governments of Germany*, 4th ed. (New York: Thomas Y. Crowell, 1975), p. 131.

16. See James Q. Wilson, *Political Organizations* (New York: Basic Books, 1973), chap. 9; and Theodore Marmor, Donald Wittman, and Thomas Heagy, "The Politics of Medical Inflation," *Journal of Health Politics, Policy and Law* 1 (Spring 1976): 69–81.

17. Kassenärztliche Bundesvereinigung, "Stellungnahme zum Regierungsentwurf eines Krankenversicherungs-Kostendämpfungsgesetz, Köln, n.d., mimeo, p. 1.

18. "Das Geschäft mit der Krankheit," *Der Speigel* 26, nos. 11, 12, 13 (1972).

19. *Der Spiegel, supra*, chap. 5, note 36, p. 66.

20. Ibid., p. 70.

21. Ibid., p. 68.

22. Kassenärztliche Bundesvereinigung, *supra*, note 17, p. 4.

23. "Ärztestreik: 'Der Staat wird erpresst,'" *Der Speigel* 31, no. 8, (1977): 21–24.

24. *Der Spiegel, supra*, chap. 5, note 36, pp. 62, 70.

Chapter Ten

1. For a fascinating exploration of this topic, see Daniel Bell, *The Coming of Post-Industrial Society* (New York: Basic Books, 1973). Also Don K. Price, *The Scientific Estate* (Cambridge, MA: Harvard University Press, 1965).

2. Grant McConnell, *Private Power and American Democracy* (New York: Random House, Vintage Books, 1970).

3. Ibid., pp. 142–46.

4. See Mario Bognanno, James B. Dworkin, and Omotayo Fashoyin, "Physicians' and Dentists' Bargaining Organizations: A Preliminary Look," *Monthly Labor Review* (June 1975) pp. 33–35; Richard D. Lyons, "Unions for Doctors Are Growing Trend," *New York Times*, June 18, 1972, p. 1; Philip R. Alper, ed., *Doctors Unions and Collective Bargaining: Report of Proceedings* (Berkeley: University of California, Institute of Industrial Relations, 1974); and James A. Reynolds, "Is the Doctor Union Movement Dead?" *Medical Economics* 53 (23 August 1976): 140–59.

5. Social Security Amendments of 1972, *U.S. Code*, vol. 42, sec. 1320c (suppl. 2, 1972).

6. U.S. Senate, Finance Committee, *Social Security Amendments of*

1972, S. Report 92–1230 to accompany H.R. 1, 92d Congress, 2d sess., 1972, pp. 154–269.

7. *U.S. Code*, vol. 42, sec. 1320c–1(b) (suppl. 2, 1972).

8. For a more detailed description of medical care foundations, see Richard H. Egdahl, "Foundations for Medical Care," *New England Journal of Medicine* 288 (March 8, 1973): 491–98.

9. But there are also cases where an established peer review foundation dominated by the state medical society was *not* able to secure designation as the PSRO for its area, such as the North Carolina Medical Peer Review Foundation.

10. *U.S. Code*, vol. 42, sec. 1320c–5(a) (suppl. 2, 1972).

11. PSROs have the authority to conduct several types of review to accomplish these objectives: they are supposed to provide certification of all elective admissions to hospitals; they are to certify emergency admissions to hospitals; and they are to provide concurrent certification for continuing care once a patient has already been treated in a hospital.

12. *U.S. Code, supra*, note 10.

13. Peter Rosenberg, "Kostendämpfung in der GKV kein gesundheitspolitisches Ruhekissen," *Sozialer Fortschritt* 27 (1978); 161.

14. Clark C. Havighurst and James F. Blumstein, "Coping with Quality/Cost Trade-offs in Medical Care: The Role of PSROs," *Northwestern University Law Review* 70 (1975): 41.

15. For an excellent discussion of the legislative history of PSROs and the shift from cost containment to quality assurance objectives during the implementation phase, see ibid., pp. 38–45.

16. See Herder-Dorneich, *supra*, chap. 5, note 19, pp. 290–91; and William A. Glaser, *Paying the Doctor: Systems of Remuneration and Their Effects* (Baltimore: Johns Hopkins University Press, 1970), pp. 157–59.

17. Victor Fuchs, "The Growing Demand for Medical Care," in Fuchs, ed., *supra*, chap. 1, note 15, p. 66.

18. Robert H. Brook and Francis Appel, "Quality of Care Assessment: Choosing a Method for Peer Review," *New England Journal of Medicine* 288 (1973): 1323–29.

19. For a consideration of the potential impact of PSROs on one kind of nonmajority practice, the health maintenance organization, see Clark C. Havighurst and Randall Bovbjerg, "Professional Standards Review Organizations: Are They Compatible?" *Utah Law Review* (Summer 1975): 381–421.

20. See, for example, Paul M. Ellwood, Jr., et al., "Health Maintenance Strategy," *Medical Care* 9 (May-June 1971): 291 ff; and Clark C. Havighurst, "Health Maintenance Organizations and the Market for Health Services," *Law and Contemporary Problems* 35 (Autumn 1970) pt. 2: 716–95.

21. Health Maintenance Organization Act of 1973, *U.S. Code*, vol. 42, sec. 300e (Suppl. 3, 1973). For a more detailed political history of the health maintenance organization strategy, see Paul Starr, "The Undelivered Health System," *The Public Interest*, no. 42 (1976), pp. 64–85.

22. Starr, *supra*, note 21, p. 75.

23. For a review of such studies through 1972, see Milton I. Roemer and William Shonick, "HMO Performance: The Recent Evidence," *Milbank Memorial Fund Quarterly: Health and Society* 51 (Summer 1973):

271–317. For a more recent evaluation, see Clifton Gaus, Barbara Cooper, and Constance Hirschman, "Contrast in HMO and Fee-for-Service Performance," *Social Security Bulletin* 39 (1976): 3–14; and Harold S. Luft, "How Do Health Maintenance Organizations Achieve Their 'Savings'?" *New England Journal of Medicine* 298 (June 15, 1978): 1336–43.

24. *Health Services Information*, August 11, 1975, p. 1 (newsletter of Interstudy Institute for Interdisciplinary Studies, Minneapolis, MN).

25. Merwyn Greenlick, "The Impact of Prepaid Group Practice on American Medical Care: A Critical Evaluation," *Annals of the American Academy of Political and Social Science* 399 (January 1972): 100–113.

26. Milton I. Roemer, et al., *Health Insurance Effects: Services, Expenditures, and Attitudes under Three Types of Plans* (Ann Arbor: University of Michigan School of Public Health, 1973).

27. Greer Williams, *The Kaiser-Permanente Health Plan: Why It Works* (Oakland,Calif.: Henry J. Kaiser Foundation, 1971), p. 40.

28. California Council for Health Plan Alternatives, "Feelings About the Kaiser Foundation Health Plan on the Part of Northern California Carpenters and Their Families" (Burlingame, Calif., 1973), cited in Judy Carnoy, Lee Coffee, and Linda Koo, "Corporate Medicine: The Kaiser Health Plan," *Health-PAC Bulletin*, no. 55 (1973), pp. 4–18.

29. See Roemer and Shonick, *supra*, note 23, p. 293, for a review of several studies; also the findings of David M. Kessner and Carolyn E. Kalk, *Contrasts in Health Status*, vol. 2: *A Strategy for Evaluating Health Services* (Washington, D.C.: Institute of Medicine, National Academy of Sciences, 1973); and Luft, *supra*, note 23, pp. 1336–43.

30. Howard Waitzkin, "Latent Functions of the Sick Role in Various Institutional Settings," *Social Science and Medicine* 5 (1971): 63.

31. See Comprehensive National Health Insurance Act of 1974, S. 2970, 93d Congress, 2d sess., February 6, 1974.

32. See Alain Enthoven, "Consumer Choice Health Plan," *New England Journal of Medicine* 298 (1978), 2 pts.: 650–59 and 709–20.

33. Ibid.

The following bibliography is intended to aid people who wish to inquire further into the German health care system. Because comprehensive bibliographies on professionalism and on American health policy are available elsewhere, materials on these two topics were omitted. The references are divided into English and German publications, in order to provide a ready list for those who do not read German.

Publications in English

Altenstetter, Christa. *Health Policy-Making and Administration in West Germany and the United States*. Beverly Hills: Sage Publications, 1974.

Altenstetter, Christa. "Planning for Health Facilities in the United States and West Germany." *Milbank Memorial Fund Quarterly/Health and Society* 51 (1973): 41–71.

Eichhorn, Siegfried. "German Federal Republic." In Douglas-Wilson, I., and McLachlan, Gordon, eds., *Health Services Prospects: An International Survey*. pp. 81–98. Boston: Little Brown, 1973.

Glaser, William A. *Health Insurance Bargaining*. New York: Gardner, 1978.

Glaser, William A. *Paying the Doctor: Systems of Remuneration and Their Effects*. Baltimore: Johns Hopkins University Press, 1970.

MacLeod, Gordon. "National Health Insurance in the Federal Republic of Germany and Its Implications for U.S. Consumers." *Public Health Reports* 91 (1976): 343–48.

Pflanz, Manfred. "German Health Insurance: The Evolution and Current Problems of the Pioneer System." *International Journal of Health Services* 1 (1971): 315–30.

Pflanz, Manfred, and Geissler, Ulrich. "Rapid Cost Expansion in the Health Care System of the Federal Republic of Germany." *Preventive Medicine* 6 (1977): 290–301.

Reinhardt, Uwe. "Health Costs and Expenditures in the Federal Republic of Germany and the United States." In Teh-Wei Hu, ed., *International Health Costs and Expenditures*, DHEW Publication No. NIH 76–1067, pp. 249–290. Washington, D.C.: U.S. Department of Health Education and Welfare, 1976.

Rimlinger, Gaston V. *Welfare Policy and Industrialization in Europe, America, and Russia*. New York: Wiley, 1971.

Safran, William. *Veto-Group Politics: The Case of Health Insurance Reform in West Germany*. San Francisco: Chandler, 1967.

Stone, Deborah. "Health Care Cost Containment in West Germany." *Journal of Health Politics, Policy and Law* 4 (1979): 176–99.

Stone, Deborah. "Professionalism and Accountability: Controlling Health Services in the United States and West Germany," *Journal of Health Politics, Policy, and Law* 2 (1977): 32–47.

Von Haunalter, George, and Chandler, Virginia. "Health Care Expenditures in Four Western European Countries." SRI Business Intelligence Program. Research Report No. 606. Menlo Park, CA: Stanford Research Institute, 1978.

Publications in German

Auerbach, Walter. "Doppelstandard in der medizinischen Versorgung?"

Sozialer Fortschritt 21, no. 2 (1972): 36–38.

Bauer, E. "Krankenkassen und Vertrauensärztlicher Dienst." *Arbeitsmedizin Sozialmedizin Arbeitshygiene*, no. 1 (1968), pp. 19–21.

Bogs, Walter, et al. *Soziale Sicherung in der BRD: Bericht der Sozialenquête-Kommission.* Stuttgart: Kohlhammer, 1966.

Bundesministerium für Arbeit und Sozialordnung. *Eine stabile Rentenversicherung und eine gesunde Krankenversicherung.* Bonn, 1977.

Bundesministerium für Jugend, Familie, und Gesundheit. *Gesundheitsbericht.* Bonn und Stuttgart: Kohlhammer, 1971.

Deutscher Bundestag. 6. Wahlperiode. *Bericht über die Erfahrungen mit der Begutachtung der Arbeitsunfähigkeit durch den Vertrauensärztlichen Dienst (VäD) und über das Zusammenwirken der Kassenärzte (Kassenzahnärzte), der Krankenkassen, und des VäD.* Drucksache VI/3200. Bonn, February 23, 1972

Deutscher Bundestag. 7. Wahlperiode. *Bericht der Bundesregierung über die Erfahrungen mit der Einführung von Maßnahmen zur Früherkennug von Krankheiten als Pflichtleistungen der Krankenkassen sowie den zusätzlich von den Krankenkassen gewährten Maßnahmen der Vorsorgehilfe.* Drucksache 7/454. Bonn, April 5, 1973.

Ferber, Christian von. *Gesundheit und Gesellschaft: Haben wir eine Gesundheitspolitik?* Stuttgart: Kohlhammer, 1971

Ferber, Christian von. *Sozialpolitik in der Wohlstandsgesellschaft.* Hamburg: Wegner, 1967.

Gehb, Klaus. "Die ärztliche Versorgung in der Bundesrepublik Deutschland." *Deutsches Ärzteblatt-Ärztliche Mitteilung* 74 (1977): 1351–59.

Gesellschaft für Sozialen Fortschritt e.V. *Der Wandel der Stellung des Arztes im Einkommensgefüge.* Bonn, 1974.

Günther, Sven. "Beeinflussung des Krankenstandes durch den Vertrauensärztlichen Dienst." *Bundesarbeitsblatt* 14 (1963): 431–33.

Griesewell, Gunnar. "Strategien der Kostendämpfung in der sozialen Krankenversicherung." Pts. 1 and 2. *Sozialer Fortschritt* 26 (1977); 84–89, 110–12.

Hadrich, J. *Arzthonorar und Morbidität in der sozialen Krankenversicherung.* Berlin: Duncker und Humblot, 1957.

Hartwig, Hans. "Das Lohnfortzahlungsgesetz und der Vertrauensärztliche Dienst." Pts. 1 and 2. *Soziale Sicherheit* (1971); 293–95, 332–34.

Hartwig, Hans. "Aufgaben des Vertrauensärztlichen Dienstes." *Die Ortskrankenkasse* 52 (1970): 568–75.

Heeke, August. "Die Uberwachung der Wirtschaftlichkeit in der Kassenärztlichen Versorgung," *Die Ortskrankenkasse* 47 (1965): 577–78.

Herder-Dorneich, Philipp. *Analyse der Gesetzlichen Krankenversicherung: Drei Untersuchungen.* Berlin: Erich Schmidt, 1965.

Herder-Dorneich, Philipp. *Sozialökonomischer Grundriß der Gesetzlichen Krankenversicherung.* Cologne: Kohlhammer, 1966.

Heinemann, Gustav W.; Liebold, Rolf; and Heinemann, Peter J. *Kassenarztrecht auf Grund der gesetzlichen Bestimmungen und der Rechtsprechung.* 4th ed. Vol. 1. Berlin and Wiesbaden: Engel, 1973.

Institut für angewandte Sozialforschung (INFAS). "Selbstverwaltung in der Sozialversicherung." Bonn–Bad Godesberg, July 1975.

Kastner, Fritz. "Kassenärztliche Vergütungssysteme—Pauschal- oder Einzelleistungsvergütung?" Pts. 1, 2, and 3. *Die Ortskrankenkasse* 47 (1965): 11–16, 57–61, 89–93.

Kaufmann, Franz-Xaver; Hegner, Friedhart; Hoffman, Lutz; and Krüger, Jürgen. *Zum Verhältnis zwischen Sozialversicherungsträgern und Versicherten.* Forschungsvorhaben im Auftrage des Bundesministeriums für Arbeit und Sozialordnung. Bielefeld, 1971.

Klette, Dieter. "Die Kassenarztverträge der sozialen Krankenversicherung: Ihr geschichtlicher Werdegang mit Motiven." Doctoral dissertation. Eberhard-Karls-Universität, Tübingen, 1965.

König, G. "Behandelnder Arzt und Vertrauensarzt." *Arbeitsmedizin Sozialmedizin Arbeitshygiene,* No. 1 (1968), pp. 13–15.

Kortmann, Dieter. Der Übergang von der Pauschal- zur Einzelleistungsvergütung bei der Honorierung von Kassenärztlichen Leistungen. Doctoral dissertation. Wirtschafts- und Sozialwissenschaftlichen Fakultät, Universität Köln, 1968.

Külp, Bernard. "Kontrollmechanismen innerhalb des Gesundheitswesens." In Wilfred Schreiber, ed., *Gesetzliche Krankenversicherung in einer freiheitlichen Gesellschaft,* pp. 113–32. Berlin: Erich Schmidt, 1963.

Lüth, Paul. *Niederlassung und Praxis: Eine kritische Einführung.* Stuttgart: Thieme, 1969.

Landmann, F. *Die Lösung der Kassenarztfrage.* Elberfeld: Grimpe, 1898.

Naschold, Frieder. *Kassenärzte und Krankenversicherungsreform: Zu einer Theorie der Statuspolitik.* Freiburg: Rombach, 1967.

Plaut, Theodor. *Der Gewerkschaftskampf der deutschen Ärzte.* Volkswirtschaftliche Abhandlungen der badischen Hochschulen. Heft 14. Karlsruhe: G. Braunsche, 1913.

Preller, Ludwig, *Sozialpolitik: Theoretische Ortung.* Tübingen and Zurich, 1962.

Quandt, Otto. *Die Anfänge der Bismarckschen Sozialgestzgebung.* Berlin: Ebering, 1938.

Rauskolb, Christa. *Lobby in Weiss.* Frankfurt: Europaische Verlagsantalt, 1976.

Rosenberg, Peter. "Die Finanzen der gesetzlichen Krankenversicherung." *Vierteljahreshefte zur Wirtschaftsforschung* 3 (1973): 198–201.

Rosenberg, Peter. "Gesundheitspolitik in der Krise." Deutsches Institut für Wirtschaftsforschung, *Wochenbericht* 43 (1976): 115–21.

Rosenberg, Peter. "Kontrolle der Kostenentwicklung im Gesundheitswesen." *Sozialer Fortschritt* 23 (1974): 165–68.

Rosenberg, Peter. "Kostendämpfung in der GKV kein gesundheitspolitisches Ruhekissen." *Sozialer Fortschritt* 27 (1978): 158–61.

Ruegenberg, Horst. "Perspektiven einer Weiterentwicklung der gesetzlichen Krankenversicherung." *Die Ortskrankenkasse* 58 (1976): 1–12.

Schicke, Romuald. *Arzt und Gesundheitsversorgung im gesellschaftlichen Sicherungssystem.* Freiburg: Rombach, 1971.

Schmitt, Alfred, "Medizinische Versorgung muss klassenlos sein!" *Sozialer Fortschritt* 21 (1972): 201–4.

Schmitt, Heinz. *Entstehung und Wandlungen der Zielsetzungen, der Struktur, und der Wirkungen der Berufsverbände.* Berlin: Duncker and Humblot, 1966.

Scholmer, Joseph. *Die Krankheit der Medizin.* 2d rev. ed. Darmstadt and

Neuwied: Hermann Luchterhand, 1972.

Siebeck, Theo. "Die kassenärztliche Gesamtvergütung." Pts. 1, 2, and 3. *Die Ortskrankenkasse* 47 (1965): 169–74, 204–12, 234–41.

Siebeck, Theo. *Zur Kostenentwicklung in der Krankenversicherung.* Bonn: Bundesverband der Ortskrankenkassen, 1976.

Siebeck, Theo. "Die Krankenversicherung in den 60er Jahren," Pts. 1 and 2. *Die Ortskrankenkasse* 53 (1971): 101–14, 150–61.

Siebeck, Theo. "Das Vergütungssystem im Kassenarztrecht." *Die Ortskrankenkasse* 45 (1963): 501–16.

Siebeck, Theo. "Wandlungen und Tendenzen im Kassenarztrecht." *Die Ortskrankenkasse* 53 (1972): 799–810.

Silomon, H. "Vertrauensarzt–Behandelnder Arzt." *Arbeitsmedizin Sozialmedizin Arbeitshygiene,* no. 1 (1968), pp. 16–18.

Sörenson, Thomas. "Automatisierte Laborleistungen neu bewertet." *Die Ersatzkasse,* no. 7/8 (1973), pp. 508–12.

Stirn, Hans. "Wenn Ärzte zuviel verordnen . . . Die Fragwürdigkeit der Überprüfung kassenärztlicher Praxen." *Arbeit und Sozialpolitik* 24, no. 6 (1970).

Ströer, Heinz. *Die Soziale Versicherung.* Munich: Beck, 1971.

Ublich, E. "Zur Prüfung der Wirtschaftlichkeit der kassenärztlichen Leistungen." Pts. 1 and 2. *Der Niedergelassene Arzt* (1974), pp. 11–22 and 75–88.

Voges, Friedrich. "Die aktuelle Honorarsituation der Kassenärzte." *Deutsches Ärzteblatt* 63 (1966): 2349–77.

Wekel, Wolfgang, "Änderungen des Kassenarztrechts." *Die Ortskrankenkasse* 59 (1977): 117–20.

Wirtschafts- und Sozialwissenschaftliches Institut des Deutschen Gewerkschaftsbundes GmbH. *Die Gesundheitssicherung in der Bundesrepublik Deutschland: Analyse und Vorschläge zur Reform.* 2d ed. Köln: Bund, 1971.

Wirzbach, Hans J. "Die finanzielle Sicherung der Krankenhäuser." *Arbeit und Sozialpolitik* 27 (1973): 111–14.

A Note on Publications of Executive Agencies, Bodies of Public Law, and Interest Groups.

The Bundesministerium für Arbeit und Sozialordnung (Ministry of Labor and Social Affairs), which is responsible for the entire social insurance program, publishes a wealth of useful information. Its annual Social Reports (*Sozialberichte*) describe the legislative changes in the health insurance system, present data on public expenditures for social services, and indicate the government's policy goals for the immediate future. An excellent English-language article that explains how to read the Social Reports and compares them with similar reprots of other countries is Paul Fisher, "Social Reports of the German Federal Republic, 1970–71," *Social Security Bulletin* 35 (1972): 16–29.

The ministry also publishes a special Survey of Social Insurance (*Übersicht über die soziale Sicherung*) approximately every three years. These surveys provide a descriptive overview of each social insurance program. In 1972, the ministry issued an English translation of the 1971 edition; otherwise, they are all in German.

Finally, the ministry also publishes the most authoritative and up-to-date statistics on administration and financing of health insurance in its monthly series. *Arbeits- und Sozialstatistik*.

The Bundesärztekammer or BÄK (Federal Chamber of Physicians), in Cologne, issues an annual activities report (*Tätigkeitsbericht*) summarizing new developments in health policy and articulating the chamber's position on controversial issues. The BÄK also issues occasional special position papers.

The Kassenärztliche Bundesvereinigung or KBV (Federal Association of Insurance Doctors), whose headquarters are in the same building as those of the BÄK, compiles useful data from a variety of sources in its statistical yearbooks, but these "yearbooks" are actually published only once every three or four years. The KBV has a research institute, the Zentralinstitut für die kassenärztliche Versorgung in der Bundesrepublik Deutschland, which publishes a series of special studies on selected topics in health policy.

The BÄK and KBV jointly publish a monthly journal, *Deutsches Ärzteblatt*, which includes a special section on politics and policy ("Ärtzliche Mitteilung") in each issue. In addition, there is usually a special issue of the *Deutsches Ärzteblatt* devoted to the proceedings of the annual meeting of the BÄK.

The Bundesverband der Ortskrankenkassen or BdO (Federal Association of Local Sickness Funds) in Bad Godesberg publishes a variety of useful materials. Its biweekly journal, *Die Ortskrankenkasse*, carries analytical articles, reprints of laws, regulations, and court decisions affecting health policy, and descriptions of current events in health policy, as well as statements of the BdO's position on various issues. The BdO publishes an annual business report (*Geschäftsbericht*), which highlights developments in the social insurance system during the year, as well as an annual statistical and financial report (*Statistischer und Finanzieller Bericht*). In 1976, the BdO established its own research institute, the Wissenschaftliches Institut der Ortskrankenkassen (WIdO). Its research topics include manpower resources and planning, financing of health insurance, epidemiology, and utilization of medical services and drugs, and it publishes research results in a special series of reports.

The major trade union organization, Deutsches Gewerkschaftsbund, also has a research institute, the Wirtschafts- und Sozialwissenschaftliches Institut, located in Düsseldorf, that occasionally publishes special studies on health insurance reform.